Pocket Guide to Quality Improvement in Healthcare

Reneè Roberts-Turner
Rahul K. Shah
Editors

Pocket Guide to Quality Improvement in Healthcare

Springer

Editors
Reneè Roberts-Turner
Division of Nursing
Children's National
Health System
Washington
DC
USA

Rahul K. Shah
Surgery and Pediatrics
Children's National
Health System
Washington
DC
USA

ISBN 978-3-030-70779-8 ISBN 978-3-030-70780-4 (eBook)
https://doi.org/10.1007/978-3-030-70780-4

This Springer imprint is published by the registered company Springer Nature Switzerland AG
The registered company address is: Gewerbestrasse 11, 6330 Cham, Switzerland

This book is dedicated to our patients and families.

Reneè dedicates this book to her family, husband and children, Lewis, Rhea, and Louis; her mom Bettie; and little brother Rolan: gratitude for their unwavering support and unconditional love.

Rahul dedicates this book to his wife, Banu, and children, Amir and Nishu, for their patience and understanding for the countless times their family time has been interrupted to care for someone else's child/family.

Preface

We are excited to present this book, *QI on the Fly*. We are healthcare clinicians, healthcare leaders, healthcare executives, and, most importantly, we are children, parents, siblings, friends, neighbors, co-workers, and patients ourselves. This book is for everyone mentioned, and more. We are interested in creating a resource inclusive of every healthcare stakeholder that conveys the foundations of healthcare quality and can be referenced often. The existing literature and books on this subject are too formal – consisting of hundreds of pages, and delving into theoretical considerations and case vignettes.

How is a newly appointed board member to their community hospital expected to learn healthcare quality and safety rapidly? How does a parent whose child is being admitted to a hospital quickly learn the "in's and out's" of how a healthcare organization to ensure their child receives the best care? How is a newly graduated clinician prioritizing onboarding with human resources, obtaining their licensure, learning their new role, and overlaying the understanding quality improvement on top of this? How does a nurse influence a patient care issue resulting in an exceptional outcome? It is inconceivable to imagine one being able to process and assimilate these myriad demands.

QI on the Fly is written for anyone with a vested interest in quality improvement; *QI on the Fly* is essentially written for all of us. *QI on the Fly* is for everyone that wants to know more about quality improvement and how quality improvement processes and data impact healthcare outcomes – for others and themselves.

A landscape of the existing offerings for quality improvement and safety reveals an absence of easily digestible material based on the reader's role. It's almost a given that an individual patient or family, someone working in healthcare, a healthcare executive, or a board member will read the chapter pertinent to their specific role; however, we hope that these stakeholders will not stop there. Each chapter is constructed to stand on its own and be rapidly read and digested. This book aims to provide a broad overview of quality improvement concepts and how they can be immediately pertinent to one's role. This book intends to give an immediate understanding and whet one's appetite for the quality improvement cycle. If you are still hungry after reading the high-level information, there are many textbooks that go deep into each of the topics introduced. Thank you for giving us the privilege of your interest and attention while reading *QI on the Fly*.

Washington, DC, USA

Reneè Roberts-Turner
Rahul K. Shah

Acknowledgments

We take a moment to acknowledge the "giants upon whose shoulders we stand upon." We have learned so much from our mentors that provided us the unique opportunity to be leaders within our fields. Ultimately, we appreciate the patience of our patients and families. With gratitude, Reneè and Rahul

Contents

Contributors

Eric Manuel Balmir Children's National Hospital, Washington, DC, USA

Sopnil Neil Bhattarai Department of Performance Improvement, Children's National Hospital, Washington, DC, USA

Stephanie Borinsky Department of Pediatrics, Eastern Virginia Medical School, Norfolk, VA, USA

Sharon Bostic Nurse Consultant, Upper Marlboro, MD, USA

Jessica A. Cronin Division of Anesthesiology, Pain, and Perioperative Medicine, Children's National Hospital, Washington, DC, USA

Jeffrey N. Doucette Thomas Jefferson University Hospitals, Philadelphia, PA, USA

Amy C. Drader Growth Partners Consulting, Washington, DC, USA

Lisbeth D. Fahey Quality Improvement & Safety, Children's National Hospital, Washington, DC, USA

Ana Figueroa-Altmann Department Patient Safety Officer, Children's Hospital of Philadelphia, Philadelphia, PA, USA

Alia Fink Performance Improvement Department, Children's National Hospital, Washington, DC, USA

Sandip A. Godambe Department of Quality and Safety and Division of Pediatric Emergency Medicine, Children's Hospital of The King's Daughters Health System, Norfolk, VA, USA

Department of Pediatrics, Eastern Virginia Medical School, Norfolk, VA, USA

Maya S. Godambe Department of Pediatrics, Eastern Virginia Medical School, Norfolk, VA, USA

Gen Guanci Cultures of Excellence, Creative Health Care Management, Bloomington, NM, USA

Jessica Herstek Department of Pediatrics, The George Washington University School of Medicine and Health Sciences, Children's National Hospital, Washington, DC, USA

Tina Kunze Humbel Clinical Nurse Manager, Baltimore, MD, USA

Jeffrey Li Independent Researcher, Clarksville, MD, USA

Robert C. Lloyd Institute of Healthcare Improvement, Boston, MA, USA

Nikolas Mantasas Children's National Hospital, Washington, DC, USA

Layla San Martin University of Maryland Medical System, Baltimore, MD, USA

Janice J. Mason Department of Nursing Science, Professional Practice & Quality, Children's National Hospital, Washington, DC, USA

Kathryn Merkeley Children's National Hospital, Washington, DC, USA

Asha S. Payne, MD, MPH Children's National Hospital, Washington, DC, USA

Srijaya K. Reddy Department of Anesthesiology, Division of Pediatric Anesthesiology, Monroe Carell Jr. Children's Hospital/Vanderbilt University Medical Center, Nashville, TN, USA

Reneè Roberts-Turner Division of Nursing, Children's National Health System, Washington, DC, USA

Rahul K. Shah Chief Quality and Safety Officer, Children's National Hospital, Washington, DC, USA

Eric Shelov Department of Biomedical & Health Informatics, Division of General Pediatrics, Perelman School of Medicine, University of Pennsylvania, Children's Hospital of Philadelphia, Philadelphia, PA, USA

Xiaoyan Song Office of Infection Control/Epidemiology, Children's National Hospital, Washington, DC, USA

Fabienne L. Vastey New York-Presbyterian Brooklyn Methodist Hospital, Brooklyn, NY, USA

Heather Walsh, MSN, RN, PCNS, BC Children's National Hospital, Washington, DC, USA

Katherine M. Worten Quality, Safety, and Analytics, Children's National Hospital, Washington, DC, USA

1 An Introduction to Quality Improvement: What We Need to Know in Healthcare

Reneè Roberts-Turner and Rahul K. Shah

This book is for you! Healthcare is one of the most complex endeavors where there is only one successful outcome: optimal care for the patient. All efforts and strategies in healthcare should be focused on solely one thing: the patient. How do we ensure the delivery of the highest level of quality in a safe manner? *It is not easy.*

A patient may encounter only a nurse, a therapist, and a provider (all referred to as the "sharp end" of care delivery) and not necessarily interact with the environmental services team, the finance team, the dietary team, etc. (sometimes referred to as the "blunt end" of care delivery); however, for a successful outcome with the highest level of care delivery in the safest manner, all

R. Roberts-Turner (✉)
Nursing Science, Professional Practice, Quality and Magnet® Program Director, Children's National Hospital,
Washington, DC, USA
e-mail: rrturner@childrensnational.org

R. K. Shah
Chief Quality and Safety Officer, Children's National Hospital,
Washington, DC, USA
e-mail: rshah@childrensnational.org

R. Roberts-Turner, R. K. Shah (eds.), *Pocket Guide to Quality Improvement in Healthcare*,
https://doi.org/10.1007/978-3-030-70780-4_1

parts of the healthcare team have to be working together all the time. *It is not easy.*

We (Reneè and Rahul) are both part of the sharp end of care delivery as a nurse and surgeon, respectively. We are both part of the blunt end of care delivery as part of the administrative leadership of Children's National Hospital, a tertiary-care freestanding children's hospital in Washington, District of Columbia, in the United States. Our hospital has been serving patients for 150 years! The reader can imagine the tremendous change that has occurred during that time in care delivery. One thing has remained solid and constant: we serve the patients.

To best serve our patients, we have to continually look for innovative approaches to drive care delivery, within the framework of safe and quality care. We do this by learning from other industries, other hospitals, and the overall academic literature. We take known strategies and implement these to improve care. In doing so, we quickly realized that we are missing an opportunity to educate colleagues, support staff, board members, and, ultimately, patients. There is not a definitive primer for all those involved in healthcare to be on the same page. How can we expect a patient and their family to understand PDSA cycles and how the model for improvement is being utilized to ensure she receives the highest level and safest care? How can we expect a board member, who has the fiduciary responsibility to serve the community's interests and ensure their hospital's success and to learn about the safety and quality part of the organization when they must be focused on the financials, strategy, and the hospital's role in the community? This book fills this gap. This book provides all different parts of the healthcare system a primer on safety and quality so that we can speak a common language and jointly drive safety and quality care for our patients.

The objectives of this book are to help all healthcare professionals understand the basic principles of quality improvement by walking the reader through the step-by-step quality improvement process, as well as through the various domains that comprise the parts of the quality and safety engine. We hope to be able to guide individuals and organizations to fully engage staff in quality improvement. This knowledge for all healthcare staff is necessary, as healthcare systems must continue to strengthen and fortify care delivery and the desired associated outcomes. We aim to educate individuals that want to know more about quality improvement and how QI processes and data impact the care provided to patients and families. To achieve this goal, we lay out the foundations of healthcare quality and describe how these methodologies can be applied to the everyday work habits of the healthcare professional in their settings. In addition, we provide patient and family perspectives and relevant quality improvement information for decision making entities such as management and guidance for governance from hospital boards.

A framework is necessary to understand healthcare in this era and, subsequently, how to utilize quality improvement tools and techniques. The Donabedian triad is a commonly used improvement framework and the one we both employ all the time in our organization! The triad is structure, process, and outcomes.

We focus and perseverate on the structure – do we have the right teams, are the correct individuals on the team, does the team meet frequently enough, does the team have a clear reporting hierarchy, etc.

Then we ensure the processes are in place – are there audits, do we track metrics, how do we respond when data goes the wrong direction, etc. By spending over 95% of our team's time and effort on structure and processes, outcomes are expected to follow.

A fallacy in quality improvement is to go right for the outcome without consideration of the structure and processes that need to be in place for the outcome to be resulted and then sustained.

The ultimate aim is to create a high-reliability organization. High-reliability organizations (HROs) "operate under very trying conditions all the time and yet manage to have fewer than their fair share of accidents [1]." Achieving the outcomes in the goal would be the holy grail of care delivery; as a patient, I want this and expect it. As a healthcare system, we owe it to our patients and community to strive for reliability. Weick and Sutcliffe's easy-to-read book [1] has become mantra in healthcare organizations that strive to deliver optimal and safe care using their high-reliability principles. Behaviors associated with high-reliability organizations include preoccupation with failure, sensitivity to operations, reluctance to simplify interpretations, deference to expertise, and commitment to resilience [1]. These are absolutely nonnegotiable tenets in a healthcare setting and deserve highlighting. *Preoccupation with failure* involves a culture that encourages the identification of work processes that raise concern for potential failure [1]. *Sensitivity to operations* requires an awareness of how processes and systems affect the organization through early recognition of threats to the organization, which involves attentiveness to small changes in daily work [1]. *Reluctance to simplify* requires identification of the slight differences between threats through in-depth scrutiny, which involves using various methods of exploration, designed to identify the real source of the problem [1]. *Deference to expertise* requires that decision making is directed towards the person with the most knowledge and expertise to handle the situation at hand, usually not the top of the organization [1]. *Commitment to resilience* requires that everyone is confident regarding the organization and that it will "bounce back" from any events that inevitably will occur [1].

Events will occur. We have to have systems in place that can predict to the best of our ability when these events will occur and then put in place measures to control the events and any future events. This is what high-reliability organizations do – day in and day out. *It is not easy.*

The ultimate goal of the quality improvement process, conceptually, is to implement interventions to make iterative improvements to a process or system and sustain change. The process begins by identifying a process or system that may be inefficient, and hence we begin to identify existing problems. Hospital executives, leaders, frontline staff, and patients and families can all help to identify inefficient quality and safety processes. Identifying the problem involves recognizing mistakes and identifying when there are too many steps in the process or when a process is too complicated; ultimately, a process or system that does not produce reliable results is amenable to a quality improvement intervention. Not all problems are amenable to an improvement initiative. Categories of potential projects usually address one or more of the following: effectiveness, efficiency, patient satisfaction, safety, throughput, waste reduction, provider, and staff engagement.

The questions asked to identify the problem can differ depending on if you are attempting to fix or design your system or process. When looking to fix a current system or process, answering the following questions can help you identify the problem:

What worries you? What makes you believe there is an easier way to get the expected outcomes? Are we "working hard and not smart"? Are we failing to meet practice standards? Have we defined the standard work?

When you are seeking to design a new system or process, answering the following questions can help you identify the problem: Is there an opportunity to utilize work that we are already doing? In what areas are we not the best, in comparison to similar institutions? What can we do better?

Additional questions to consider when identifying the actual problem include the following: What were your thoughts at the time you decided this was a problem? Why is this a problem? How does this problem affect the quality of patient care? Does this problem affect efficiency, effectiveness, equity, timeliness of care, family centeredness, or safety of care provided? These are the six domains of healthcare quality as defined by the Institute for Healthcare of Improvement. Placing the potential improvement initiative into one of the six domains of healthcare quality further confirms the need to address the problem and helps the management and the board to understand the prioritization of the initiative. This information also can assist in scoping or identifying the specificity of the problem. Indeed, chapters in this book will demonstrate how, ultimately, a data-driven approach will identify opportunities for improvement and assist in measuring improvement.

What is most important is that projects are aligned with organizational goals and priorities. Aligning improvement projects with organizational goals ensures hospital leadership support, minimizes "roadblocks," and improves the accessibility to available resources.

Before starting a project, determining if the organization or clinical area is ready to embark on such a project can help determine success and is a compulsory assessment. When organizational or clinical area readiness is high, organizational members are more likely to initiate change, exert significant effort, exhibit greater persistence, and display cooperative behavior [2]. Members of the organization/unit must be committed to the change by having a shared desire to implement a change and also believe that capacity for the change to occur exists. The ability to implement change is directly related to the organizational/unit member's perception of three key determinants: task demands, resource availability, and situational factors [2].

Specifying metrics is necessary to make the problem measurable and explains what is needed to make actual improvements. A popular quote by Dr. Donald Berwick, founder of the Institute for Healthcare Improvement and past CMS Administrator, is "[S]ome is not a number. Soon is not a time." Indeed, the specificity requisite in a quality improvement project will ensure proper processes are developed to drive the desired change with outcomes expected to follow.

We discuss various models for improvement and strategies to embark on improvement initiatives in this book, with the goal for the reader to understand potential techniques or methodologies that can be employed to drive and sustain change. At Children's National, we employ the Institute for Healthcare Model for Improvement, which utilizes aim statements and key driver diagrams to identify, prioritize, and be the levers of change. There are many sources of deep knowledge on these techniques, and the goal of this book is to provide the reader with a general awareness that these principles exist and how they should be utilized in your healthcare setting to drive improvement. This textbook is not meant to be a thorough or exhaustive tome on these important topics.

Ultimately, a project will need a robust aim statement, which should include data and numeric goals that can be reliably measured. A common mnemonic is to develop a SMART aim: one that is "S"pecific, "M"easurable, "A"pplicable, "R"ealistic, and "T"imely. The aim statement must include what the project will increase or decrease, the group or population the project will affect, the baseline (from what) and goal (to what), and a timeframe (accomplish by when and sustain for how long).

The SMART aim should be linked to a global aim. In other words, SMART aims should be part of larger organizational goals rather than be siloed to be most impactful. We provide an example of a blank key driver diagram (Fig. 1.1) that is used at Children's National Hospital. The template facilitates a shared, common understanding and alignment throughout the organization and provides instant recognition for management, leadership, and the board to instantly understand a quality improvement initiative. It is imperative to maintain that the global aim is the larger picture – what we are trying to improve.

With a SMART aim and a global aim, we have to ask what are the levers that will result in improvement. These are called drivers, and the primary drivers are often referred to as key drivers. Ultimately, the key driver diagram (Fig. 1.1) is the road map to help achieve a shared understanding of what we are trying to

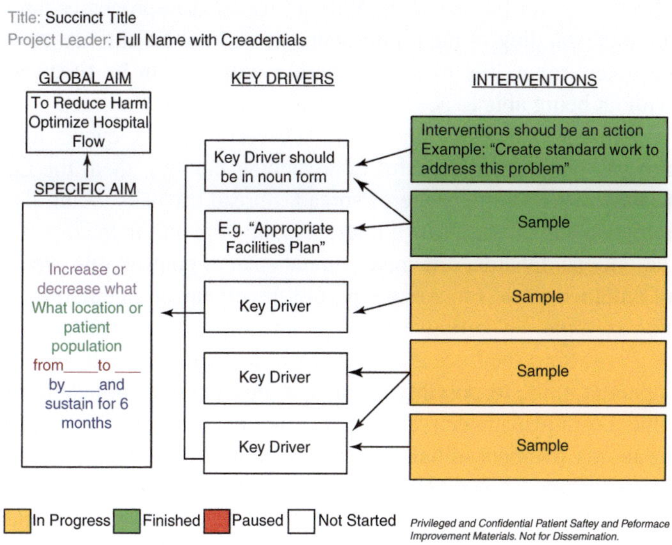

Fig. 1.1 Key driver diagram template used at Children's National Hospital

achieve and how we are going to get to the specific goal. A key driver diagram is not static. As conditions change, drivers are accomplished, and milestones are achieved, it is necessary to update the project key driver diagram. Management and the board can assist the organization by framing questions and guiding decisions and tactics based off the key driver diagram.

Once we have identified a problem that is amenable to an improvement methodology, and we have created a SMART aim with the KDD (key driver diagram), then we can begin the "hard" work. This book details cycles for improvement, which are called PDSA cycles and are iterative, narrowly scoped, improvement initiatives. As we progress through several PDSA cycles, conducted in serial and parallel fashion, we must monitor performance. There is a primer on data in this book that barely touches the level of sophistication of data that healthcare organizations use to measure and describe the data associated with improvement. We employ at least a dozen of individuals committed to using data to drive improvement! The data helps tell the story, but also to monitor performance. Without robust data processes, and an understanding of data, improvement will not be attained as it becomes impossible to know where a project is in its lifecycle without being able to accurately measure it; data is the ruler.

We will eventually determine successful PDSA cycles and drivers which are successful in advancing the aim; then, the QI project moves to the stage of spread. Spread involves taking the initiative and project from a micro-system (one unit in the organization, one division, one management span of control, one group of employees, etc.) to a larger part of the organization/enterprise. For example, an initiative that was successful in a specific unit (e.g., 4-Main) then needs to be spread, as pertinent, to the other inpatient units, to possibly outpatient areas, and if applicable to other hospitals/care delivery sites in your organization. The spread of an improvement initiative can happen quickly or over a longer period of time, depending on the process that needs to be in place to support the change. Management and the board can provide tremendous assistance in the important decision and guidance as to when to spread successful initiatives.

The final stage of a QI initiative is the sustainment of gains. This is probably the most difficult part of the project. When does a project no longer require day-to-day management and oversight and when can we trust that the structure and processes that we have put into place will be able to be sustained as a permanent change to the processes? This is a very difficult decision, as prematurely putting a project into sustain mode or delaying too long to put a project into sustain mode comes at an opportunity cost. Resources and time are finite; if a project is ready to be sustained, then doing so supports reallocation of efforts to new initiatives or those that need additional support. However, prematurely sustaining a project can be more harmful than the initiative itself. Your hospital's chief quality and safety leader, chief medical or nursing officer, or other leaders and managers can help best assist with framing this discussion and assisting with this determination driven by deference to expertise.

The easy part of this work is getting started. This book is intended to remove the intimidation factor of quality, safety, quality improvement, and change. As a primer, we hope that readers will be able to quickly understand key concepts that will provide a ladder for each reader to climb in their journey of quality improvement sophistication. At the conclusion of reading this book, the reader will have the tools to engage in meaningful discussions with patients, colleagues, management, and the board on various facets of quality improvement. *It is this easy.*

References

1. Weick KE, Sutcliffe KM. Managing the unexpected: resilient performance in an age of uncertainty. 2nd ed. San Francisco: Jossey-Bass; 2011.
2. Bryan J, Weiner A. Theory of organizational readiness for change. Implement Sci. 2009;4:67.

Model for Improvements 2

Katherine M. Worten

Improvement Science

Every successful project starts with a plan. Whether it be a house project to build and design the perfect outdoor space, a history project for school, or a business project for work, those that are well defined from beginning to end have a higher rate of success. While hard work is most certainly a contributor, the real driver is the method or planning applied to tackle the issues at hand.

Taking a systematic approach to addressing a problem in order to achieve desired outcomes is not just a strategy, but a scientific method.

The science of improvement, as defined by the Institute for Healthcare Improvement (IHI), is "an applied science that emphasizes innovation, rapid-cycle testing…and spread in order to generate learning about what changes… produce improvements" [1].

Improvement science is not a new concept and has been around for a while with organizations like Toyota and Bell Labs [2]. The gurus of quality improvement (QI), Walter Shewhart, W. Edwards Deming, and Joseph Juran, simplified and refined the science of

K. M. Worten (✉)
Quality, Safety, and Analytics, Children's National Hospital, Washington, DC, USA

R. Roberts-Turner, R. K. Shah (eds.), *Pocket Guide to Quality Improvement in Healthcare*,
https://doi.org/10.1007/978-3-030-70780-4_2

improvement. While studying the method these leaders used to improve the process for building better cars or improving information technology and communication, the question became whether or not this same philosophy and attitude could be translated to other industries. Luckily for health care, the answer was a resounding "yes!"

The Associates of Process Improvement (API) defines the science of improvement and further explains that the proper application of this science requires the integration of improvement methods, tools, and subject matter experts to develop, test, implement, and spread changes [3]. In health care, there are a variety of approaches or models used to foster improvement, efficiency, and effectiveness of a system or a process. A couple of models used in health care QI are the Model for Improvement (MFI) and lean/Six Sigma. While it's important to choose a reliable model to guide your work efforts, it is more important that you trust the process and fully commit to using the QI tools and processes.

Model for Improvement

The Model for Improvement (Fig. 2.1), developed by API, has been successfully used in hundreds of health care organizations across the globe [3] to improve diverse processes and outcomes. The model has two parts: answering three fundamental questions and conducting tests of change. By answering the three fundamental questions, you have established your plan of action. The questions that are required to be answered by collaborative teams are the following: (1) What are we trying to accomplish? (2) How will we know that a change is an improvement? (3) What change can we make that will result in improvement? The second part to the Model for Improvement is implementing and testing change through what is called the Plan-Do-Study-Act (PDSA) cycle (Fig. 2.2).

Question one, "What are we trying to accomplish?," speaks to the end goal or aim. In other words, "why are we here?" This might seem like an easy question, but to do this right, there must

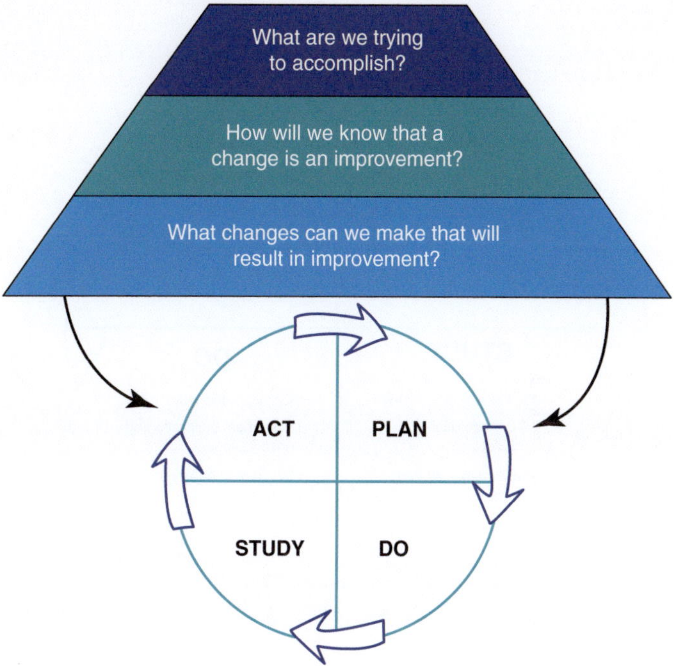

Fig. 2.1 The Model for Improvement

be a level of specificity provided to the answer, including the population that will be affected and the time frame which one would wish to achieve their accomplishment. By providing specific details, you have delivered clear and specific intent among your team. Everyone will be on the same page and have a clear understanding of the goal and hold each other accountable for getting the job done.

Question two is, "how will we know that a change is an improvement?" or "what does *good* look like?" Teams should use quantitative measures and data to identify measures that track their success. Where is the finish line? Once a team reaches that measure, this is the point at which you might trigger the "we did it!" celebrations. An important thing to consider is a realistic target or goal that is deemed successful. Will you be able to eliminate

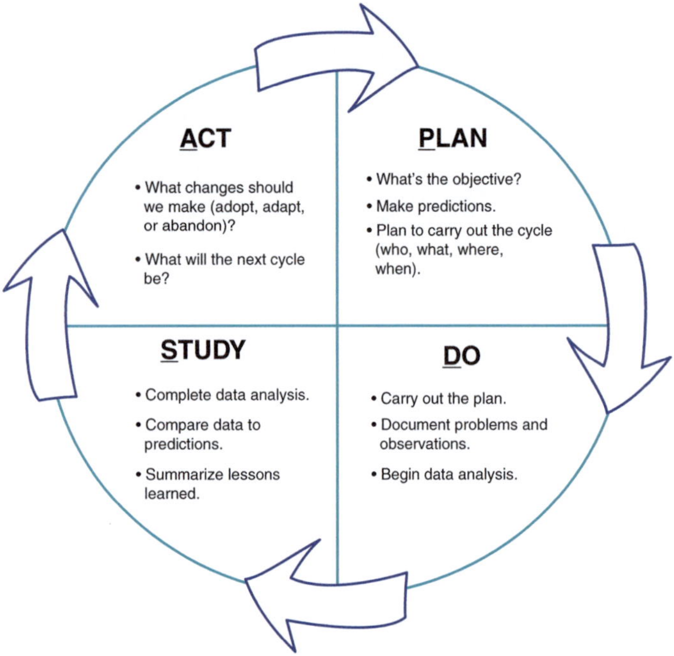

Fig. 2.2 Plan-Do-Study-Act (PDSA) cycle

patient wait time in a clinic schedule by 90% in 6 months' time? Probably not, and that's okay! Setting realistic goals will help your team visualize the finish line and have it within reach. The emphasis is on incremental change and incremental improvement. You can shoot for a 20% improvement over 6 months and maybe another 15% improvement another 6 months after that.

Question three asks, "what change can we make that will result in improvement?" This is when innovation, creativity, and sometimes common sense come into play. The team, who should consist of those who are closest to the work, generates ideas and solutions they think will positively impact change. It is important to know there is not one right answer. There is no silver bullet that will solve the entirety of a problem identified in a system or process. Teams should select a number of changes they think will bring them closer to success.

It might be easy to simply identify the aim/goal, determine quantitative measures for success, and come up with solutions that we believe would lead to improvement. But then what? The key ideas and solutions developed are then implemented in a cyclical fashion, which leads us to the second critical component that makes up the Model for Improvement. The concept of the Plan-Do-Study-Act (PDSA) cycle is to test out changes to see if they are helping or hurting. To put this into perspective, you wouldn't buy a car fresh off the conveyor belt without having the breaks, airbags, and steering tested. Automakers use a series of tests to make sure their final product will satisfy their customers, both in comfort and safety and reliability. The idea behind testing a car is that it allows manufacturers to work out the kinks. Potential problems that negatively impact the product can be corrected or modified slightly before the car goes into full production or rolls onto a dealership lot. If you think about it from a cost perspective, it is a lot cheaper to eliminate a problem before production, rather than having to find and fix the problems after the fact.

The PDSA cycle asks that teams take their solutions (the plan), try it (do), observe the results (study), and then do something with that plan based on what you learn (act). If you have favorable results, you can *adopt* the intervention. If the test of change sort of worked, you can *adapt* the idea or tweak it a little and try again. And if you have failed miserably, it's okay to abandon the idea altogether. The PDSA cycle allows for a threshold of failure. It is at such a small scale that the idea of failing, learning from the failure, and trying again is part of the process.

Rather than trying to boil the ocean and solve world peace in one fell swoop, teams are encouraged to make incremental, small-scale improvements. The idea is to start small with hunches, theories, and ideas and discover what works and what doesn't work. From there, iterative changes and refinements are made with each cycle until you find the sweet spot that results in improvement. This will organically create a ramp of multiple PDSA cycles of improvements shown in Fig. 2.3.

Let's take a real-world example to demonstrate how to apply the Model for Improvement in the scenario of moving to a new city or even a different part of town. Typically a new move requires

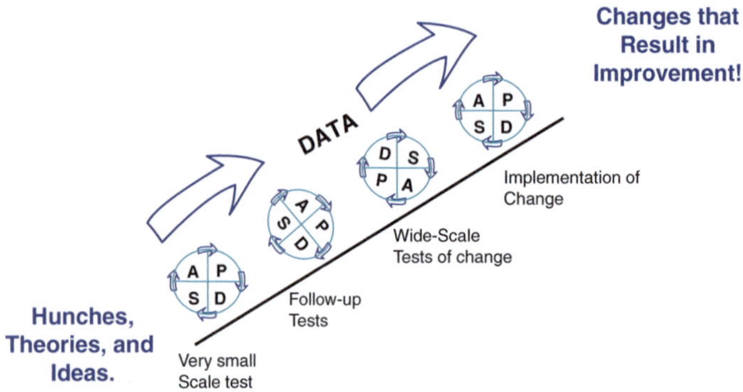

Fig. 2.3 Multiple PDSA cycles

a bit of time to become acclimated with your surroundings. For me, it starts with finding the nearest essentials: grocery stores (fingers crossed for a Trader Joe's), pharmacy, coffee shops, and of course, Target. In addition, I need to make sure I know how to get to and from work the most efficient and safest way possible. My goal or aim was to get to work no later than 7:30 am Monday to Friday each week while maximizing sleep. I started timing myself each day to gather data about how long it was taking me to get to work in the morning. Without knowing this information, it would be impossible for me to set a goal or to know what good, better, and best might look like. After 1 month, or 20 days, I had an average time of arrival of 14 minutes, the quickest time was 11 minutes from A to B, and the longest time was 18 minutes. Going back to our Model for Improvement, the goal or aim was set, the measures of success were defined by the data I had collected, and now, I got to explore ideas and decide what changes I could try to achieve my results. The first thing I did was to consult the experts to the process who could have already found solutions to the very problem I was trying to solve. More often than not, you can assume that someone at some point in time has attempted to address the very problem you are trying to tackle. In that case, there is no need to recreate the wheel, but learn what successes and failures they experienced. I could find someone that lived nearby and traveled to the same location and ask what route they take and why. I could also do a little research and see what Google Maps had to offer. I found there were three routes to get me from point A to B, two taking the highway and one taking back roads. Based on the information gathered, I would start my first PDSA cycle: the route. I decided to take the highway with the shortest estimated time of arrival, according to Google Maps, a new way from the baseline data I had gathered. After testing that out for a couple of days, I learned that it took me closer to 15 minutes to my destination. I decided to tweak my plan just slightly by taking the same route, but leaving 5 minutes earlier; this would be my second PDSA cycle. I made my plan, left 5 minutes earlier the next couple of days, and studied my results, and since they were favorable, I decided to adopt that practice to leave at the same time to avoid the traffic I had experienced when leaving a bit later. Once I had achieved my goal of getting to work by 7:30 am every day by standardizing the time I left and the route I took, I could say that that the results were a success.

The Model for Improvement demonstrates how defining, measuring, and making continuous changes are key to learning and accelerating improvement efforts. It is much more than deciding *what* you are going to do, but *how* you are going to do it and *why*.

Lean/Six Sigma

It wasn't more than 2 years into my career as a Project Associate in the Project Management Department, when I was asked to help coordinate logistics for a consulting group who would be conducting a 5-day "Lean" training for a number of hospital leaders. One of the perks of this task, besides the unlimited supply of coffee, was that I was able to participate and complete the training program myself. The concepts and tools that I learned from this methodology were the jump-off point for finding my niche with process improvement. It was simple and translatable from one industry to the next, and I became more and more eager to study and practice the methodology in health care. Lean management principles have been used effectively in manufacturing companies for decades, and similar to the Model for Improvement, it is another model for that has been successfully applied to the health care setting. In simple terms, "lean thinking" is using less, to do more, or making the right work easier to do. This model takes a close look at processes from start to finish and aims to drive out waste to optimize and maximize productivity and value, all from the customer's perspective. "lean thinking" originated in Japan and was hugely successful and most well known in the Toyota Production System [6].

While a health care setting might not come close to resembling the operations of a factory, surprisingly, the concepts of lean lend itself nicely to both industries while it focuses on streamlining processes, reducing cost, and improving quality and timely delivery of products and services. The key concepts in lean include *leadership*, *culture*, and *process*.

Introducing lean thinking in an organization is not a simple task. It requires a great deal of *leadership* support and cannot be done in a disjointed fashion. A strong commitment and support is required from the top leadership as well as engagement from middle management and frontline staff to think differently and view their work from a completely different lens – the lens of the customer or, in health care, the patient [4].

Alongside the support and leadership of the Executive Team, *culture* is another key component of building a lean organization. Tools and techniques are implemented but only successful if lean thinking is woven into the fabric of the organization. An organization's culture sets the beliefs and values that its people follow. The challenge of accepting a culture built on lean principles is accepting that your work and the systems that you work are not perfect. This is particularly challenging for health care professionals who pride themselves on the precise work they do day in and day out. Admitting or recognizing that your daily tasks are wasteful and do not add value can be a difficult realization to admit out loud. However, a nurse may not see that searching for supplies that are not readily available is seen as waste. Although they are doing it with the patient in mind, they are unable to provide timely care because they were unable to obtain what they need when they needed it. That was seen as something that could be prevented or eliminated completely if stocked appropriately. Lean helps to understand that things such as this are not what health care professionals went to nursing school or medical school to do. They are, and at many times, underutilized when their day-to-day work requires unnecessary tasks that are considered non-value-added. Leaders are needed to help staff embrace lean practices by working together with frontline staff to flatten the hierarchies that exist within an organization to move the dial together.

The third key concept of lean considers *process*. When asked who the "customers" are in health care, you might think the answer would be those who drive the processes within a health care system – physicians, nurses, insurers, and government and insurance payers. From a lean philosophy, the patient is at the tip of the spear, and the processes should always be designed with them in mind. At the beginning of a quality or process improvement event, it is typical for the executive sponsor to kick-off the event by sharing words of wisdom, support, and perhaps a patient story to depict the importance of the task at hand. One of the most impactful demonstrations of this was when the emergency department physician champion placed an empty chair in the center of the room where the improvement event was taking place. The chair represented the patient. Everything we were going to do would be designed with that child in mind. When looking at a particular process, the focus revolves around creating the right value for the right patient or customer. The goal is to increase the valuable components while eliminating or reducing as much as possible the non-value-add or waste. Designing a perfect lean process not only maximizes and creates value, but it is also satisfying for people to perform, managers to manage, and customers or patients to experience.

One of the common strategies that help pulls the concepts of leadership, culture, and process together is to go to the *gemba* or where the work is done [5]. Doing this provides a level of understanding and appreciation for the complexities and challenges while also highlighting the best practices that exist in a process. Dr. David Munch, an executive from the lean training and consulting organization I received lean training from, shared the motto "go see, ask why, show respect." There was no better way to learn than from those who are doing the work in the very environment in which they do so. A fresh eyes perspective and a simple conversation may be all that is needed to provide a robust understanding of the challenges at hand. People learn best when they are directly involved, and leadership who practice this can make change happen very quickly.

Six Sigma

If you've heard of lean, you might have heard that model coupled with Six Sigma. While lean works to drive out waste, Six Sigma focuses on reducing variation within a process to help drive teams to create stable, reliable systems [7]. Similar to other quality methods, Six Sigma appreciates and promotes a systematic approach starting with identifying the problem and ending with implementing solutions. In Six Sigma, this is called DMAIC for Define, Measure, Analyze, Improve, and Control the improvement.

Six Sigma views processes with a statistical focus. The philosophical perspective of Six Sigma says that processes require inputs and produces outputs. If you control what you put in to a process, you can control what you get out of one. Using data and statistical process control (SPC) charts, you can easily see the variation that exists in a process and how your interventions can contribute to reducing variation further, creating a more predictable and manageable process.

In Fig. 2.4, you can see the ideal bell-shaped or normal distribution curve. The area under the normal distribution curve makes up six standard deviations (sigma) away from the center (three in each direction) which is where the name Six Sigma comes from.

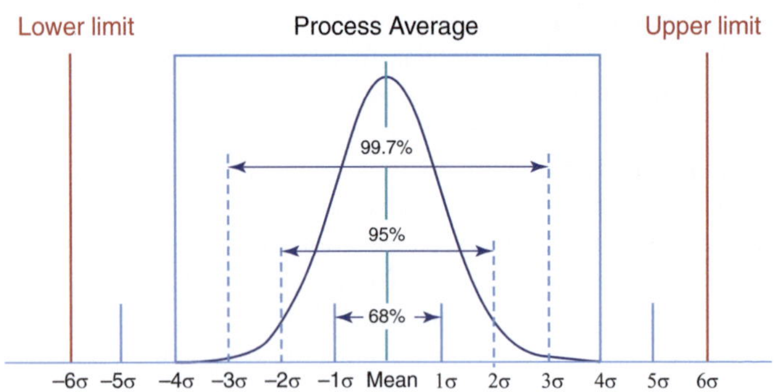

Fig. 2.4 Six Sigma quality performance

Moving one standard deviation each direction away from the graph's center (2 sigma) covers 68.2% of the data. Two standard deviations in either direction (4 sigma) cover 95.4% of the data, and three standard deviations (6 sigma) cover roughly 99.7% of the data. That's saying that 99.7% of the data points will consist of outputs with zero defects or errors. In statistical terms, Six Sigma quality performance means there are 3.4 defects for every million opportunities [7].

Six Sigma is broad and complex, so if you followed nothing in the paragraph above, the key takeaway is to imagine Six Sigma as a quality control program. When your process data falls within six standard deviations, it is normal variation that is inherient to any process. Anything that falls outside six standard deviations warrants investigation. The smaller or tighter the variation, the more realible or predictable your process.

Lean and Six Sigma were originally two separate business philosophies to optimize processes, both providing customers with the best possible quality, cost, delivery, and safe flexibility. Today most industries combine the two methodologies. The "sweet spot" for Lean and Six Sigma is to use them as one method together to achieve excellence in quality and operations. While lean in general is about making processes more simple, Six Sigma is about the quality of what you deliver. Lean/Six Sigma is a data-driven and fact-based model of improvement that values preventing defects opposed to detecting defects. The customer-focused approach is driven by reducing variation and driving out waste all while fostering enhanced process standardization.

Why Should You Care?

In a 1990s interview with Steve Jobs, he talks about core principles of quality improvement. He explains that "In most companies, if you're new and you ask 'why is it done this way?' the answer is, 'because that's the way we do it here.' The largest contribution to much of this quality thinking is to approach these ways of doing things… scientifically" [8]. Methodologies such as Lean, Six Sigma, and the Model for Improvement are the mechanisms or the approach to help us identify why we do what we do. By using data-driven decision-making, we are able to see where to focus our efforts and subsequently measure and monitor improvement.

Every one of us will encounter the need to use the health care system. At one such encounter, you may have been asked by a health care professional to change your personal practice in order to improve your health. Changing your personal practice might mean doing something more or something less to see positive results. If we ask our patients to change personal practice to improve, one might argue that patients deserve the same from the health care system.

Whether you are a frontline health care worker, health care executive, board member, or anyone who encounters the system, it is important to have a basic understanding of the methodologies and science of improvement to identify opportunity and help drive change. Being an active learner and participant with improving systems and processes that you experience firsthand will result in being part of the solution. Improving the performance in the health care environment can help produce reliable, cost-effective processes while improving care delivery and patient outcomes. This ever-evolving industry requires a constant need to challenge the status quo and seek opportunities to improve on behalf of your patients, your family, and your community.

References

1. Langley GJ, Moen RD, Nolan KM, Nolan TW, Norman CL, Provost LP. The improvement guide: a practical approach to enhancing organizational performance. 2nd ed. San Francisco: Jossey-Bass Publishers; 2009.
2. Aguayo R. Dr Deming: the American who taught the Japanese about quality. London: Mercury Books; 1991.
3. Associates in Process Improvement. 2020. apiweb.org. Accessed 20 June 2020.
4. Deming WE. The new economics for industry, government, and education. Cambridge, MA: The MIT Press; 2000.
5. Smith B. Lean and Six Sigma: a one-two punch. Qual Prog. 2003;36(4).
6. Going Lean in Health Care. IHI Innovation Series white paper. Cambridge, MA: Institute for Healthcare Improvement; 2005.
7. American Society for Quality. 2020. ASQ. https://asq.org/quality-resources/six-sigma. Accessed 26 June 2020.
8. Steve Jobs on Joseph Juran and Quality. WoodsEnd, Inc., & G. Howland Blackiston.

3 Measuring to Improve in Quality Improvement

Sopnil Neil Bhattarai

We have heard the phrase, "That which cannot be measured cannot be improved" often attributed to Peter Drucker, the inventor of modern business management. Drucker is considered one of the greatest management thinkers of all time [1], and his lessons about measurement can be applied to quality improvement (QI). In QI, measures serve as pulse checks in a system, based on which a healthcare practitioner can understand how the system is performing. The Model for Improvement asks, "How will we know a change is an improvement?," and this is where measures come into place. There are three main measure types: (1) outcome, (2) process, and (3) balancing. Before we look at measures, we need to understand how measures provide context, and for this, we look at the Donabedian model of care.

S. N. Bhattarai (✉)
Department of Performance Improvement, Children's National Hospital, Washington, DC, USA
e-mail: Sbhattara2@childrensnational.org

R. Roberts-Turner, R. K. Shah (eds.), *Pocket Guide to Quality Improvement in Healthcare*,
https://doi.org/10.1007/978-3-030-70780-4_3

Donabedian Model of Care

Avedis Donabedian was a health systems researcher in the University of Michigan. He is considered the founder of the study of quality in healthcare and medical outcomes research. He is most famous for creating the "Donabedian model" of care [2]. There are other frameworks that exist to improve quality, such as the Bamako Initiative and the World Health Organization framework. The Bamako Initiative focuses on economical ways of defining quality of care, such as focus on effectiveness, efficiency, sustainability, and equity. The World Health Organization framework of quality of care focuses on a philosophical understanding that high-quality healthcare is a universal right. The Donabedian model works on a macroscopic and organization and health systems level. The Donabedian quality-of-care framework states that the impact on health status is directly driven by the structure of the health system and the processes in the form of good medical practices.

How Are Structure and Processes Associated with Outcomes?

Jake Shimabukuro is an American ukulele virtuoso, and his rendition of the Beatles' "While My Guitar Gently Weeps" catapulted his career and brought ukulele into the forefront of Millennial and Gen Z pop cultures. One cannot go past 100 music videos on YouTube without encountering a ukulele cover of a song.

The ukulele is a simple string instrument belonging to the lute family. It generally has four nylon strings and fits nicely into a child's hand. Less intimidating than a six-string guitar, the ukulele is a great first instrument to pick up for anyone. I first encountered Jake Shimabukuro's tenor ukulele late 2006 and thought it was incredible. Between many years of following Jake's career, and countless YouTube ukulele stars coming out, I never actually picked up the instrument. Eleven years later, however, I finally concluded it was time. Consider my ukulele journey as self-improvement.

In 2017, my wife went to a 7-day conference, and I had my apartment for myself. After cleaning every inch, organizing all paperwork, and completing all my chores, I finally ran out of excuses. It was time. I looked for a ukulele on Craigslist and found one for a reasonable price. This simple act of starting up and actually getting the instrument was establishing the *structure*.

Without the structure, there is no context. Without the ukulele, I could not start learning the instrument. Sure, I could watch YouTube videos, but without actually picking up and trying the instrument, it would be a futile task. In healthcare, similarly, the structure is how a particular improvement journey starts.

If a hospital wants to look at the rates of *Clostridioides difficile (C. diff)*, there needs to be context where this improvement work is done. This includes the physical facility, equipment, and human resources. Without a laboratory that can test for *C. diff*, it would be a Himalayan task for the hospital to look at its rates. Without staff that could process the samples, the hospital would need another way; for example, it would need to figure out how to contract out the lab samples. The structure also involves the organization's characteristics, such as staff training. If none of the staff members trained to draw lab samples, the hospital's desire to conduct the improvement work is futile.

Structure can also be establishing systems for improvement work. Just because I picked up my ukulele does not mean that I would become a virtuoso overnight. I signed up for courses online that would provide me with some fundamentals and decided I would practice in the mornings so that I do not disturb my neighbors. In our lab analogy, the "time" could be the time allocated during leadership meetings to discuss the project. It could be venues, such as grand rounds or lectures, where individuals working on the project can report out regularly. Hospitals with established quality outcomes meetings have avenues that can help facilitate discussion of the project.

Donabedian Triad

When taken with the context of measurements, the Donabedian triad depicted in Fig. 3.1 makes perfect sense. The triad has two main bases: structure and process with the apex of the triad as the outcome. The structure and process hence hold up the outcomes. With active venues to discuss project or conduct project improvement activities, appropriate investment in equipment and training (structure), and processes actively engaged in improvement, outcomes will follow. A hospital cannot improve *C. diff* rates without investing in structure.

Outcome Measures

The outcome measure refers to your overall goal or aim. My short-term aim was to learn to play three chords in the ukulele by the end of the week. The outcome measure, in this case, would be

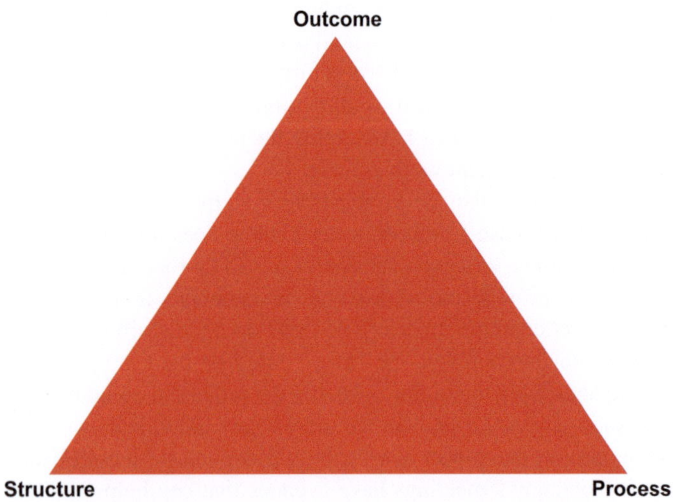

Fig. 3.1 Donabedian triad [2] sets a framework in which outcomes follow structure and processes in systems. Without the structure and processes in place for improvement activities, outcomes are tough, if not impossible, to achieve

whether I learned three chords or not based on standards that I set for myself at the beginning of the project. More discussion about these standards, also known as operational definitions, will be done later in this chapter. In a hospital setting, if you are trying to improve patient and family satisfaction in the emergency department, the outcome measure may refer to satisfaction scores. If measuring overall patient experience in the hospital, one could use a combination of outcome measures, such as health outcomes (morbidity and mortality), with patient satisfaction measures. One must track outcome measures throughout the length of the project, and the sampling strategies will be different than other measures for the project. Our care team at the hospital would need to measure *C. diff* rates every month through the end of the project.

Process Measures

When trying to make system changes, it is helpful to look at the system as a whole. However, a system does not work in isolation. It is essentially a sum of parts working together. An organ system is a network of tissues working together towards the common function. A factory is a system that produces a product. A hospital system works towards improving the healthcare of its patients. In my ukulele example, the system I establish with the structure work together to give me the outcome I desire. However, is learning three chords in ukulele something that happens right away? How do I know that I am headed in the right direction? To understand this, we need to understand the lagging and leading indicators.

Outcome measures are sometimes referred to as lagging indicators. Economists often refer to lagging indicators as "any measurable or observable variable that moves or changes direction after a change has occurred in target variable of interest" [3]. Often, these have occurred after a large shift has occurred in the markets. Some famous economic lagging indicators are the average duration of unemployment, corporate profits, labor cost per unit of output, interest rates, etc. These indicators shift upwards or downwards when some significant events have already occurred. A surge in demand may increase the consumer price index in a few months after the surge has already occurred. In our healthcare example, the lagging indicator is the *C. diff* rate of the hospital. The final rates of *C. diff*, which could be the number of events normalized by the census, will not be apparent until the end of the month. A hospital's central line-associated bloodstream infection rates will not be apparent until numbers are finalized, which lags the actual event by many months.

In philosophy, there is a type of knowledge called "a posteriori," which is knowledge that is known by experience. A posteriori is a form of lagging indicator – a change has already occurred, and the knowledge arrives afterward. Process measures are the opposite. Process measures can be referred to as leading indicators. Leading indicators are factors that change before the rest of the economy begins to go in a particular direction [4]. Market observers and policymakers predict significant changes in the economy based on leading indicators. In philosophy, process measures can be referred to as "a priori," which is knowledge that appeared beforehand, often by reasoning. In my ukulele example, a process measure is an indication of how well I may do in achieving my goals of learning three chords. Process measures help you measure how well your system is functioning to achieve your goals ultimately. In the ukulele example, it would be how often I practice. If I set up a structure (buy a ukulele, sign up for classes, etc.), I will not automatically be proficient in the instrument. I will have to practice in frequent intervals. If I slack and do not practice for a few months, my progress may be diminished. A lack of practice could be an early sign of system failure.

Similarly, in a healthcare setting, a lack of proper antibiotic prescription patterns may give a clue on why patients are developing *C diff* infections. If a hospital has a protocol, but no way of measuring how the protocol is being followed, i.e., how practitioners are adhering to the *process*, the only signal they would know would be their infection rates. Similarly, if the hospital conducts interventions, such as policy and procedure changes, education, changes to the electronic health system, etc., how would one be able to discern that the practices are changing? If education was effective, and compliance to using new guidelines is high, there is a high chance that the outcomes will follow. Process measures are a key pillar to the Donabedian framework and serve as pulse checks on how the system is working; thus, it could predict how the system performs in the future.

Balancing Measure

Balancing measures serve as the quantification of unintended consequences in the system. It is important to monitor balancing measures because iterative changes in one part of the system could affect other parts of the system and ultimately could lead to changes in other outcome measures. If a hospital wants to reduce the time patients spend in the recovery room after surgery, leaders should make sure the rates of patients returning to the surgery are not high. In the ukulele example, a balancing measure could be tracking time spent doing other activities. Normally, I work out in the mornings. If playing the ukulele reduces my time working out, this is a negative impact on my overall lifestyle. However, a word of caution: balancing measures do not always have to be negatively impacting the system. A change in the system leads to an increase in patient satisfaction but also impacts staff satisfaction in a positive manner. In this case, increased satisfaction is "good." Balancing measures are not inherently good or bad.

Operational Definitions

Operational definitions are one of the tenets of quality improvement. If the measurement is not consistent, it is impossible to say whether change over time has occurred. Here are the four rules of operational definitions [5].

1. Gives communicable meaning to the concept.
2. Specifies measurement methods and equipment.
3. Identifies criteria (inclusion vs. exclusion).
4. Has clear and unambiguous wording.

Consider the following example. Hospital-acquired C. diff rates are measured over time as infections per 1000 days of therapy. Days of therapy is a measurement that adds every day that patients are on antibiotics for a time period normalized by 1000. When coming up an operational definition for this measure, you will have to address all points: "we will measure monthly C. diff rates per 1000 days of therapy (concept) in our hospital (inclusion criteria) using CDC criteria (method)."

Data

Healthcare data is a complex topic, and this chapter will only highlight the most important concepts. For detailed discussions on data and how it is used for improvement, I highly recommend *The Health Care Data Guide: Learning from Data for Improvement* [6] by Lloyd Provost and Sandra Murray. This book is essential for further reading.

Creating strong measures sets the stage for an effective data strategy. Data can then be turned into information. Healthcare is no different than other industries in recent times: we are inundated with data. A 2016 estimate suggested that the amount of digital data is set to exceed 1 zettabyte, of which 30% is healthcare. This data represents 30 million times the data in all books that have ever been written [7]. But without context, data becomes useless. Measures help put data into context. In quality improvement work, data shown over time is of utmost importance. Without this tracking, measurement of improvement becomes impossible. Consider Figs. 3.2, 3.3, and 3.4, where a hypothetical shipping company wants to track delays in package delivery before and after implementation of a new software system. Figure 3.2 shows that before the software system, there were a total of 9 hours of delay per package. After the new system, it looks like there were 4 hours of delay per package. This looks like an incredible 56%

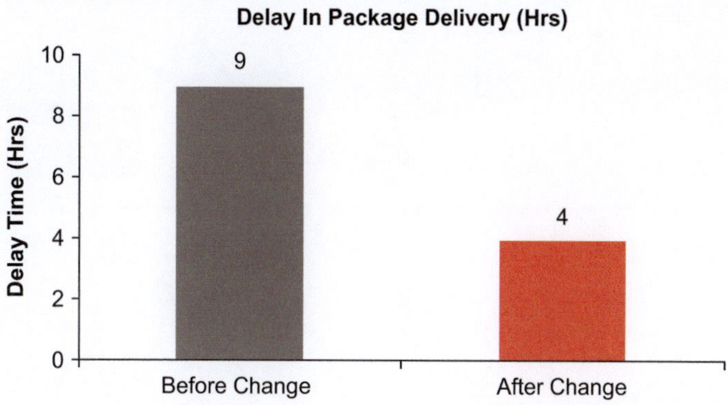

Fig. 3.2 Change is shown as pre- and post-implementation. This practice could be deceptive as they do not show sustained improvement, but rather a snapshot of "cherry-picked" data

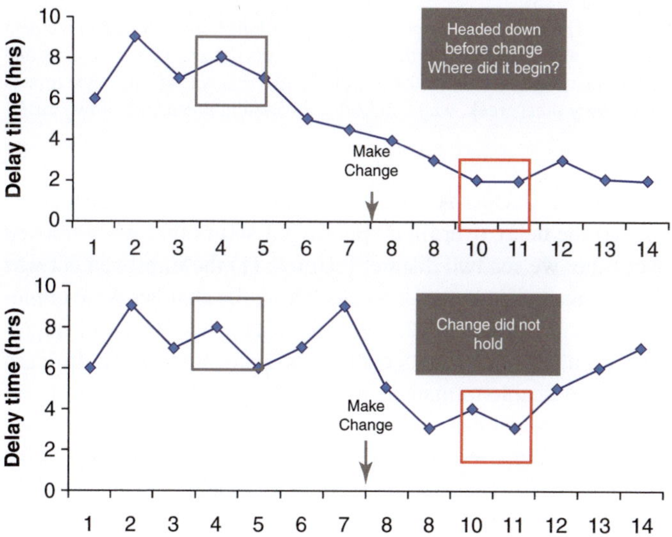

Fig. 3.3 This figure shows data over time and how changes could happen before the implementation of a new process, upon which the system leaders need to analyze whether the improvement was because of the change made or other factors. Alternatively, the lower portion of the data shows that there is an upward swing after the change, which shows sustainment did not occur

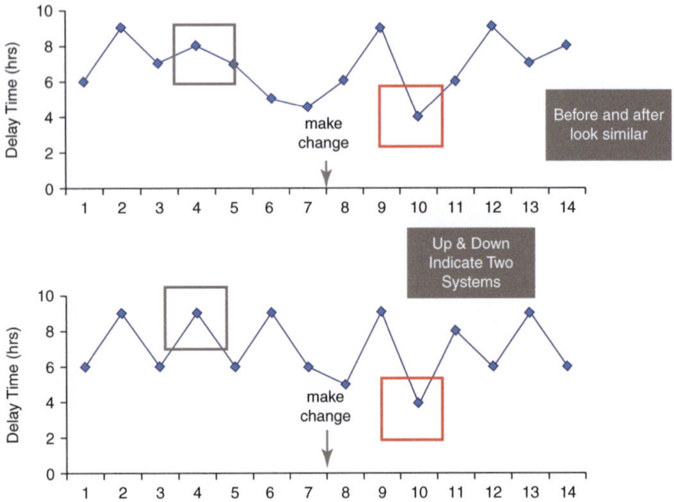

Fig. 3.4 The top image shows that before and after look similar in the data over time, which could mean that the change was not as effective. The second part of the image shows that there could be two distinct systems – the time is lower every other week, which indicates the system is reacting in two different ways

reduction in delays. However, is this the full story? What if we tracked the delay over time? Figure 3.3 shows that when tracked over time, we see two distinct features: (1) the improvement was already headed downwards weeks before the changes were implemented and (2) change did not hold after a few weeks of implementation. In both instances, the company was unable to learn and hence unable to manage nor improve. Data over time shows transparency and can show sustained changes rather than snapshots in systems. In Fig. 3.4 we see other observations: (1) the before and after change data look similar and (2) ups and downs in the data indicate that there could be two systems. When looking at data, as shown in Fig. 3.2, the company can paint the narrative that the software usage successfully decreased the shipping delays. When showing data over time, however, the data becomes more ambiguous. An ideal improvement effort shows data over time and with sustained change.

Sampling Strategies

Effective data collection has a strong sampling strategy – timing is everything. The outcome measure of a project refers to the goal of the project and should, therefore, be tracked throughout the life of the project. Process measures, if applicable to the entire project, should also span the length of the project or at least until there is sustained strong process performance. For our example of *C. diff* reduction, the rates of *C. diff* should be tracked on a regular basis based on what the team agrees upon in the beginning of the project. If the team wants to conduct a small test of change for a subset, then the subset of data should be tracked only until improvement has occurred. For example, if the team wants to track education effectiveness in new fellows, they can test a small group immediately after the education activity was implemented and then a month afterward. The data over time aspect still exists, but the sampling strategy is smaller. For any Plan-Do-Study-Act cycle, the PSDA-level data will always be smaller than the global dataset, which measures the outcome measure.

Common Data Types in Healthcare

There are two main data types in healthcare: attribute data and continuous data. Attribute data can be categorized or be assigned a characteristic. A list of patients with *C. diff* infection is an attribute. Attributes can be as small as a binary characteristic. A list of patients where the appropriateness of their antibiotic regiments is measured have two attribute characteristics: whether they received proper antibiotics ("yes") or they did not ("no").

Continuous data include data such as weight, time, and temperature. They can be measured, but they have an infinite number of possible values within a selected range. The easiest way to conceptually think about this is the idea that one cannot "count" continuous data. You would never be able to count weight, time, or temperature.

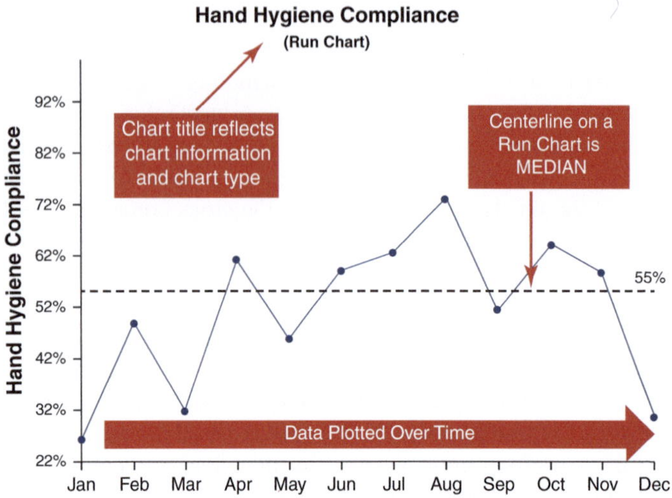

Fig. 3.5 This is a simple run chart. The data are shown over time (monthly). The central tendency or the "normal" of the data are shown as median

The type of data determines what charts one must use. This is especially important in quality improvement, where data over time are measured. The easiest way to display data over time is on a run chart. A run chart and its components are shown in Fig. 3.5. The centerline of the data is the median of all the points in the dataset. The centerline is also known as "central tendency," which means that any "middle of the road" data for the dataset will fall at or close to the median. The most common type of run chart used in healthcare is known as the control chart. A control chart is an advance mathematical chart that has complex calculations behind it. However, when properly interpreted, control charts can be extremely powerful tools for measuring hospital quality.

Basics of Control Charts

Control charts are based on the assumption that a system's data are stable. If a hospital fluctuates in its *C. diff* rates every month, there may be a need to stratify, or separate out, individual sections rather than to display the entire data as an aggregate. If the inten-

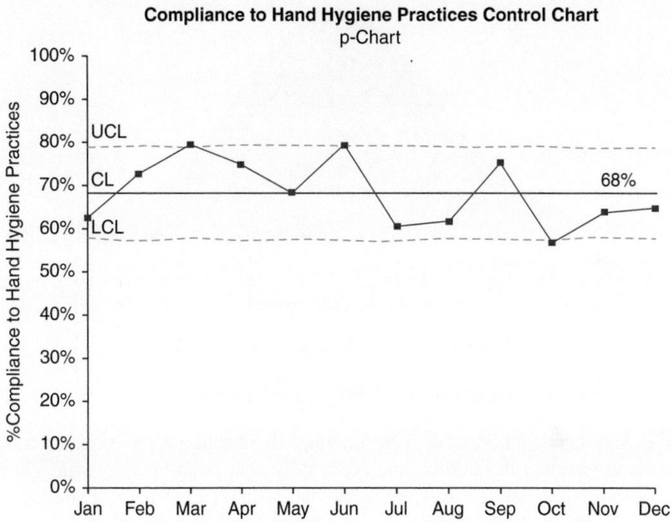

Fig. 3.6 Simple control chart. The central tendency in a control chart is the average of points. The control limits (UCL, or upper control limit, and LCL, lower control limits) fall at 3-sigma or three standard deviations from the middle

sive care units have a higher rate of *C. diff* infections, they could be pulling the central tendency of the entire system higher than usual. Control charts assume the median of the data and the average of the points are close to each other.

Control charts have thresholds known as "control limits." Control limits are based on the centerline and help project leaders decide what is "normal" for the system. Figure 3.6 shows a basic control chart. The upper control limit is three standard deviations away from the centerline.

Consider the example of men's shoe sizes. If you were to plot out men's shoe sizes, the general distribution would say that the shoe size is around 8–8.5. This becomes the central tendency, "middle of the road," or "average." On the extremes, however, there are large shoe sizes, such as size 16 or size 5. The extremes of this distribution graph can be considered as probabilities. If you were to randomly pick a man and ask them their shoe size, there is a 68% chance that they would be between 7.5 and 8.5. Similarly, the probabilities of extremely large or extremely small shoe sizes

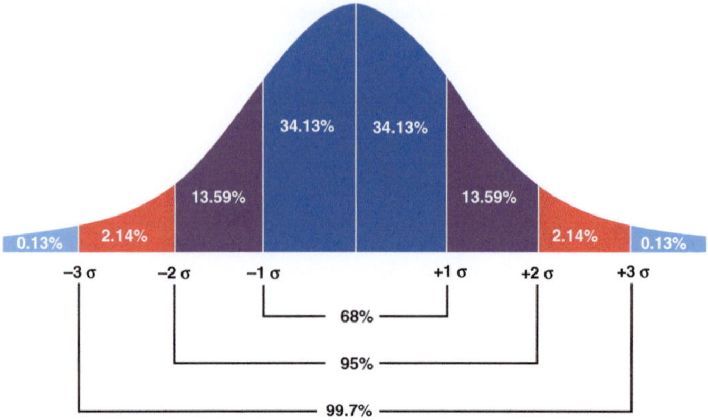

Fig. 3.7 This is a normal distribution graph divided into zones based on colors and standard deviations. The probability of a point landing within the zones is also illustrated. Any points beyond 3-sigma are considered outliers. The probability of those points is low; therefore, if they appear in the data, they must be investigated as "special cause" [8]

are fairly low. If the shoe size is size 24 or size 2, they are considered outliers, extremes, or rare events. Figure 3.7 shows a normal distribution graph.

A control chart is the same data displayed over time. The upper and lower control limits fall at three standard deviations (or 3-sigma) from the centerline. This means that if a data point is beyond 3 sigma, the probability that the data is an outlier is >99% [9]. If that data point occurs, the team must investigate and find out why that has occurred.

Control charts help us understand the concept of common cause and special cause variation. In common cause variation, the processes inherent to the system yield the result the "normal" results for the system. If I survey a normally distributed database of men for their shoe size, I should generally get the shoe size range of 7–8.5. However, what if I surveyed NBA players that are generally taller than the average population? The data would skew in the extremes. In the *C. diff* example, what if there was a dramatic increase in *C. diff* rates in the hospital and it was above the 3-sigma threshold? This would be considered a special cause variation when data behaves differently than it normally does. Special cause variations can be intended or unintended. Let us say that the team wants to improve compliance to adhering to certain protocols for antibiotics and the team implements forcing functions on the electronic medical system. Providers are unable to select any other options besides the ones chosen by the hospital committee to be the best regimen of antibiotics. This change would be considered an intentional special cause if the adherence dramatically increases beyond 3 sigma.

Special causes can also exist if data over time behave consistently away from "normal." The most common is a rule referred to as "centerline shift." A centerline shift implies that the data has deviated enough from the central tendency that the central tendency is no longer useful. Typically a centerline shift happens if eight data points are below the centerline. For example, if your commute to work is typically 45 minutes and never exceeds 1 hour, or is below 35 minutes, you could comfortably say that your average time to commute is around 45 minutes, with an upper limit of 1 hour and lower limit of 35 minutes. If all of a sudden, your commute was closer to an hour every day for 8 days in a row, one could consider that this was a shift. Your new centerline is now around an hour. Why is that the case?

If a coin is tossed once, there is a 50% probability that it is falls heads or tails. What if it falls to heads eight times in a row? You would investigate whether this coin was rigged. Similarly, if your commute was an hour instead of 45 minutes every day, there could be something special going on, such as construction or new business opening in your regular route. This example is an unintended variation and a special cause. This is a signal for improvement teams to conduct an investigation.

Control Chart Types

Control charts are based on the data that is being collected. The audience for this chapter is anyone involved in healthcare; as such, it is impossible to be able to adequately address the nuances of

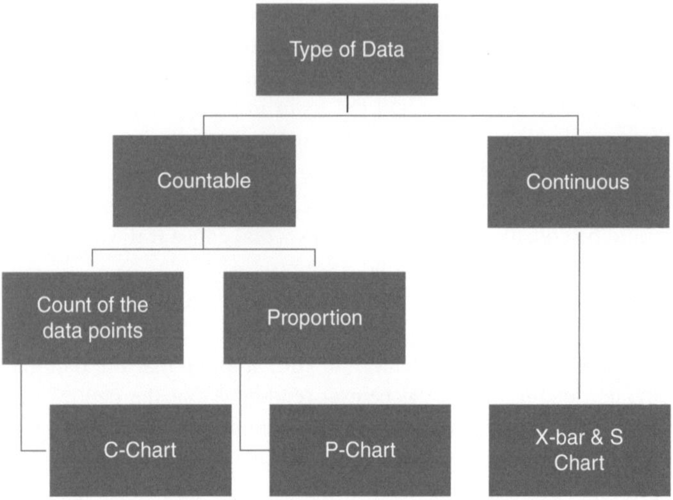

Fig. 3.8 Basic forms of control charts

control charts. The following paragraphs are simple primers to help set the stage for you to be conversant regarding control chart types.

The basic forms of control charts are shown in Fig. 3.8. The most common control chart is a c-chart, which counts data over time. These are helpful when you are just getting started with improvement work. A p-chart stands for *proportion* chart. This chart is typically utilized for compliance. If a protocol is adhered to 60% of the time, a p-chart would reflect such data.

X-charts measure the averages of continuous variables, such as times, temperature, etc. These charts take into account subtle differences between averages within a sample size. The purpose of X-charts is to show stability between points and also between sample of points. X-charts are typically used to measure average turnaround times. S-charts show the differences within standard deviations of each point. It helps users discern how points are different from each other and understand system-level nuances based on that information. If average temperatures fluctuate from 0 °F to 60 °F in 1 day, there may be system instability that an S-chart could help one determine, since the two data points are so drastically different from each other.

Putting It All Together

The Donabedian triad brings structures and processes to systems to drive desirable outcomes. Structures, processes, and outcomes should be measured, so that leaders can know when improvements lead to change. Using effective data strategies and plotting data over time, leaders can then show that their changes led to measurable improvements in their systems. Using control charts can be an effective way of displaying data over time, and the scientific basis of the control charts is digestible to anyone. Data helps us understand our system and gets us from a posteriori to a priori. The process measures tracked over time serve as leading indicators. If I am successful in learning the ukulele, it is not due to chance, but it is because I implemented structural changes and measure my processes on a continuous basis. In my case, I am no virtuoso, but I can certainly play three chords with ease, which I consider to be baby steps to a YouTube career in case quality improvement does not pan out.

References

1. Forbes. Forbes.com. [Online]; 2014 [cited 2020 June 2]. Available from: https://www.forbes.com/sites/stevedenning/2014/07/29/the-best-of-peter-drucker
2. Agency for Healthcare Research and Quality. Types of health care quality measures. [Online]; 2015 [cited 2020.10.1]. Available from: https://www.ahrq.gov/talkingquality/measures/types.html
3. Chappelow J. Investopedia. [Online]; 2020 [cited 2020 June 2]. Available from: https://www.investopedia.com/terms/l/laggingindicator.asp
4. Chen J. Investopedia. [Online]; 2020 [cited 2020 June 2]. Available from: https://www.investopedia.com/terms/l/leadingindicator.asp
5. Lloyd RC. Navigating in the turbulent sea of data: the quality measurement journey. Clin Perinatol. 2010;37(1):101–22.

6. Provost L, Murray S. The healthcare data guide: learning from data for improvement. San Francisco: Jossey-Bass; 2011.
7. Bhattarai S, RK S. Leveraging real-time data to drive quality improvement in a pediatric health system. Pediatric Investigation. 2018;2(3):184–7.
8. NIST/SEMATECH. NIST/SEMATECH e-Handbook of statistical methods. [Online]; 2012 [cited 2020.11.1]. Available from: http://www.itl.nist.gov/div898/handbook/
9. Juran JM. Juran's quality control handbook. 3rd ed. New York: McGraw-Hill; 1988.

Taking the Individual Out of the Error: Learning from the Things That Go Wrong

4

Kathryn Merkeley

Healthcare is a risky business with a high likelihood for error. Generations of healthcare workers hear the cautionary tales about the nurse who gave a lethal dose of medication or the surgeon who operated on the wrong leg. Passed along like battle stories, they serve as an ominous reminder that the stakes are high and errors happen in the most unexpected situations. Messages about following policies, filling out checklists, adhering to the standard of care, and being vigilant 100% of the time so nothing goes wrong are ingrained in every thought or action by staff. The problem is that's not quite the truth. Healthcare is a complex web of systems that must interact seamlessly to provide safe and reliable care. At the center of these complex systems are people. Well intentioned people who keep patients safe by thinking critically and making tough decisions when the stakes are high, but people are also fallible. To truly improve safety, systems must be designed to support people in doing the right thing at the right time and provide safeguards to combat human error.

K. Merkeley (✉)
Children's National Hospital, Washington, DC, USA
e-mail: kjacobsen@childrensnational.org

R. Roberts-Turner, R. K. Shah (eds.), *Pocket Guide to Quality Improvement in Healthcare*,
https://doi.org/10.1007/978-3-030-70780-4_4

Error: That Wasn't Supposed to Happen

To Err Is Human, published by the Institute of Medicine in 2000, spurred the patient safety movement of the last 20 years [1]. *To Err Is Human* challenged the belief that healthcare errors are the fault of carelss people, by highlighting the inherent risks and need for shifting response to error from a blame approach to a systems-focused, learning approach [1]. Errors are not the result of careless individuals, rather the failing of systems, poorly designed to support individuals and provide safeguards that make it easy for people to do the right thing at the right time.

People don't come to work to make a mistake, but, even at our best, we are repeatedly impacted by internal and external factors that influence our behaviors, decisions, and actions [2]. Some factors are easy to identify: fatigue, noise, or distractions. Other factors are not so readily apparent such as cognitive biases that impact decision-making or an underlying organizational culture that inhibits speaking up when something is not right. To prevent errors and patient harm, we must be aware of how these factors impact our work and design systems that alleviate the impact on our everyday performance.

Anatomy of an Error

An error means something did not go as planned or expected. What you may not know is that different types of errors, conditions, and failures contribute to safety events. To better understand how to respond to errors, it is essential to understand how they happen. Nobody is immune to error, but a basic understanding of contributing factors makes us aware of how easily and unknowingly we can succumb to the risks around us.

The term "sharp end of care" refers to individuals at the point of care who are directly interacting with patients and at the highest risk for making a mistake that causes harm [2]. When something unexpected happens, it's easy to identify the people involved and even easier to attribute the error directly to them. The blame approach disregards appreciation for the complexity of the system and other contributing factors. The real harm is missing the chance to fix breakdowns in the system that failed to stop the error from reaching the patient.

James Reason, psychologist and renowned expert on human error, coined the terms active failure and latent condition [3]. When a safety event occurs, it is actually the result of an unsafe act (active failure) intersecting with an underlying weakness in the system (latent failure), breaking down safeguards and creating the opportunity for harm [2].

Human actions and behaviors that lead to error are considered active failures [2]. Humans process a multitude of inputs, signals, and information quite efficiently and effectively. We learn from experience and store information for application at a later time. This is possible because the brain attempts to simplify information processing and decision-making into three modes: skills-based, rule-based, or knowledge-based [3]. Despite the efficiency of the human brain, errors can happen in any mode [3].

- *Knowledge-based (problem-solving mode)*: These errors occur in situations where we have no experience or rule to apply, and the response becomes a trial-and-error approach to find solutions [3].

A new nurse enters her patient's room to find him unresponsive. She is uncertain about what to do first and calls for help.

An environmental services (EVS) worker is called to clean a room in which a patient with an infectious disease is residing in. The EVS worker is uncertain of what personal protective equipment to wear, so he asks the nurse and his supervisor for help.

- *Rule-based (if-then mode)*: The brain associates a rule, generally from experience, with a situation and utilizes this information to respond appropriately [3]. Errors occur in new and unfamiliar situations for which we have no established rule to apply, the situation is misinterpreted and the wrong rule is applied (mistake), or when a rule is bypassed (violations) [3].

A new nurse enters her patient's room to find him unresponsive. She forgets to check for airway, breathing, and circulation immediately and chooses to apply the cardiac monitor as her first intervention.

The EVS worker enters the patient's room to begin cleaning. He knows he needs to use a specific disinfectant but chooses the wrong bottle from his cart.

- *Skills-based (autopilot mode)*: Skill patterns, emerging from practice and repetition, exist in our brains making it possible to carry out actions almost without thinking [3]. Errors happen when attention is taken from the task at hand by internal or external factors (slips) or steps in the process are forgotten (lapse) [3].

An experienced nurse enters the room to assist with the unresponsive patient. While preparing emergency medications, she is distracted by a question about the patient's history and prepares the wrong medication.

The EVS worker carefully cleans the patient's room per the infectious disease cleaning protocol. When he is done, he removes his personal protective equipment and heads to his next assignment. He later realizes that he forgot to review the protocol and missed a step in the cleaning process.

Understanding how the brain manages high volumes of information quickly helps us understand how errors can happen to anyone at any time. Skills-based and rule-based errors tend to be the most frequently reported as these are the most frequently utilized modes of processing [3]. This explains why it's often the people with the most experience who make the error [3]. As clinicians gain experience and knowledge, it is imperative to be aware of factors that impact our decision-making and actions such as noise or fatigue.

Violations or at-risk behavior are often referred to as "drift" or "normalized deviance," because people choose to act in a manner that misinterprets or accepts the risk associated with the action or the risk is believed to be justified in attaining the desired outcome [4–6]. Drift consists of workarounds or shortcuts used by people trying to alleviate production pressure or achieve more outcomes with fewer resources [5, 6]. The perception of associated risk diminishes over time as drift becomes a normalized and accepted practice, often passed from person to person across units and organizations [6]. Examples include nurses carrying medications for multiple patients in their pockets in an attempt to be more efficient at medication administration or physicians copying and pasting an assessment from the previous day to save time on documentation. While drift is risky, it is not intentional, and the response to errors involving drift should include an assessment of contributory external pressures and factors.

According to Reason, safety events happen when active failures intersect with latent conditions [2]. Reason developed the Swiss Cheese Model to illustrate how systems break down and safety events occur. Each layer of the cheese represents a safeguard or defense built into the system, such as technology, alerts, forcing functions, or standardization [2]. Latent conditions are vulnerabilities or holes in the system defenses (cheese) that, when triggered by an active failure or human error, allow the event to pass through the system (holes in the cheese) and reach the patient [2]. Latent conditions often lie dormant in systems for long periods or become accepted nuisances that result in workarounds or drift.

Case Study: Active and Latent Failures

A 12-year-old patient with an obvious deformity to her right arm is rushed into the emergency department waiting room by her mother after falling from her horse. The triage nurse checks the patient weight and notes a reading of 95 lbs on the scale. She quickly documents the patient's weight in the chart and takes her back to a room. An hour later, the bedside nurse is preparing ketamine for sedation and notes that the ordered dose seems very high for this patient. As the nurse double-checks the dose calculation based on the patient's weight, she notes that the chart says 95 kilograms. In her rush to take the patient to a room, the triage nurse forgot to convert the patient's weight from pounds to kilograms.

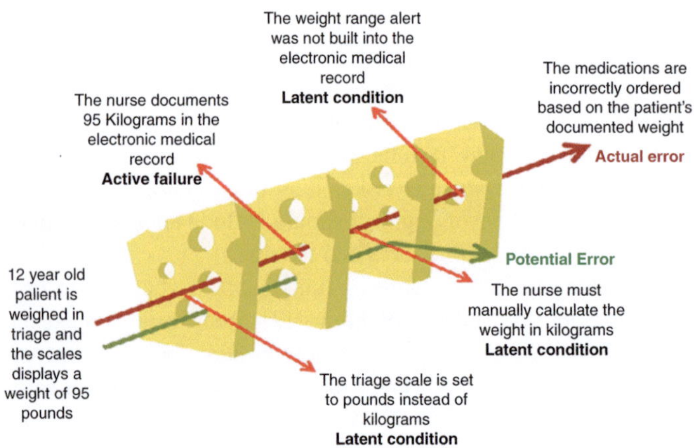

Fig. 4.1 Reason's Swiss Cheese model in action [2]

Figure 4.1 demonstrates Reason's Swiss Cheese model in action. The nurse made an error entering the patient's weight into the medical record, but the system was poorly designed to safeguard the nurse whose intention was trying to act in the best interest of the patient. According to Reason, "we cannot change the human condition; we can change the conditions under which humans work [2]." For healthcare organizations to make lasting and definitive improvements in safety, it is imperative that the response to safety events looks beyond the error of the individual and into the systems in place to support safe and reliable care.

Systems Thinking: Taking the Individual Out of the Error

> *Every system is perfectly designed to get the results it gets.* (Edward Deming [7])

Healthcare organizations are complex systems with multiple components: people, machines, technology, processes, and data functioning simultaneously to maintain operations. The continuous pipeline of new treatments, technology, and medications means healthcare of the future will be even more complex. In the course of a shift, how many people or pieces of equipment do you interact with to care for one patient? Data in the form of assessments, lab results, imaging, policies, and orders are all examples of inputs processed continuously by the human brain. Couple this with interruptions, distractions, and competing priorities, and the work of caring for patients becomes much more challenging. With so many inputs coming from, and being shared with multiple entities, it is imperative that systems are designed in a manner that supports the people at the center of the system and ensures safe and reliable care for the patients.

Case Study 3: When the System Fails Us

David is a trauma nurse with 10 years of experience working in the busiest trauma center in the city. On this night, he is the most experienced nurse on the trauma team, and it's quickly turning into a busy night. A young man comes into the trauma room with multiple broken bones and a head injury after a car accident. David works with the team to stabilize the man and prepare him for the operating room. The trauma surgeon calls for 4 mg of morphine to alleviate the man's pain. David opens the narcotic medication box to begin preparing the morphine as ordered. He's used this box so many times before that he's memorized the location of each medication. While he is reaching into the box to pull out the vial of morphine, his less-experienced colleague asks him how to apply a new type of splint to the patient's broken arm because she has never used this before. David quickly pulls up 4 mg of morphine as ordered by the physician while talking his colleague through the splinting process. David administers the morphine, and very quickly, the patient's breathing slows and his oxygenation levels drop to 60%. The team scrambles to help the patient breathe and secure his airway. When David looks back over at the vial of medication, he realizes that the vial says hydromorphone, a pain medication 7 times more potent than morphine. While answering the colleague's questions, David pulled the wrong medication from the box and administered a significant overdose of medication to the patient.

Why did the error happen? Is David at fault? How would you feel if you were in this situation? According to Reason, there are two responses to error: person-centered and systems-centered [3]. The person-centered approach focuses only on human action or decision-making that impacted the event, whereas the systems-centered approach focuses on conditions within the system that failed to safeguard against error [3]. The person-centered approach often results in a blaming or shaming response instead of addressing holes in the systems that support those at the sharp end of care [3].

Is this error David's fault? David is experienced and has given hundreds of medications to patients without incident. Using Reason's approaches to safety events, there are two ways David's leadership can respond.

Case Study 3.1: Person-Centered Approach to Error

David is called into the office by his leadership first thing the next morning. His manager demands an explanation and can't understand how someone so experienced could make this type of mistake. Before David can tell his story, the manager cuts him off, telling him this is unacceptable and he must be more vigilant in the future if he wants to keep working as a nurse here. The manager says he is lucky the patient is going to be fine and assigns David a remedial education plan to keep him from making the same mistake twice. A week later, in the staff meeting with David present, the manager talks about the event and tells the group that careless mistakes will not be tolerated. Six months later the same event happens to another experienced nurse.

Case Study 3.2: Systems-Centered Approach

David's leadership approaches him the next morning and asks how he is doing after the event and what he thinks may have happened. David states he reached into the morphine section of the box but looked back when his colleague asked a question. He's done this a million times, and he just can't believe he could make this mistake. David shows his manager the narcotic medication box in which the morphine and hydromorphone vials look the same and are stocked next to each other. Recognizing that this was a skills-based error and not the ultimate cause of the event, his manager tells him that a team will be reviewing the event to determine what the organization can do to prevent this from happening to someone else. Two weeks later, the manager reviews the findings of the analysis with staff and introduces the new layout of the medication box in which morphine and hydromorphone are stored separate from each other. The manager explains that the box's layout contributed to the error and reminds everyone to please speak up if they see vulnerabilities in the system.

Which was the more effective approach? The person-centered approach did nothing to fix the underlying problem or mitigate future harm and David was blamed in front of his colleagues. The person-centered response requires less effort, resources, and analysis but, over time, erodes the culture of safety and diminishes the likelihood of staff reporting risks or safety events in the future. Those at the sharp end of healthcare are the best resource for identifying potential risks and warding off serious events, but they will not speak up if they feel they will be blamed [4, 7]. When David's leaders took the system approach, they identified and eliminated a significant vulnerability in the equipment design. The leaders realized David wasn't the problem, and the system lacked the appropriate defenses to protect Mr. Smith. In the end, taking the easy approach to safety events causes more harm to staff, patients, and organizations.

Just Culture: Accountability Without Blame and Shame

Utilizing a system approach shifts the focus from blaming those involved and creates a nonpunitive, learning-oriented environment commonly referred to as a just culture [4]. Just culture organizations view errors as opportunities for definitive, system-level improvements. [7]. Taking the human out of the error helps reduces the likelihood to blame or shame the individuals involved and demonstrates a commitment to creating safe and reliable systems, which results in a workforce willing to speak up when something is wrong.

Just culture is not a blame-free environment without accountability for individual behaviors and actions. A just culture is a system of accountability in which leaders hold themselves accountable for creating safe systems and adequately prepare staff to do their work. In contrast, employees hold themselves accountable for their behaviors, actions, and speaking up for safety [4, 6, 7]. Organizations are employing just culture principles, and performance-based analyses actually strengthen culture because every individual recognizes his or her role in supporting the system and resulting outcomes [7].

There are numerous performance analysis guides for just culture to assist leaders in identifying and responding to human error, at-risk behaviors (drift), and reckless behavior. It is essential that organizations choose a standardized guide to ensure a consistent and equitable response. Using a standardized, performance-based decision-making guide aids leaders in how to address safety events in a manner that matches the action or behavior (Table 4.1) [4].

A just culture of accountability not only guides the response to safety events but also fosters a culture in which staff is empowered to speak up, identify risks, share ideas, and take ownership

Table 4.1 Just culture decision-making adapted from Paine (2015) [4]

Error/ behavior	Definition	Response	Example
Human error	Unintentional, honest mistakes, or active failures that result from flaws in the current system design	Learning approach to understanding the system and fixing weaknesses	A paramedic connects the oxygen tubing to the suction port because the attachment ports are the same
At-risk behavior	Unintentional risk-taking (drift or violations) where risk is not recognized or is considered to be justified based on performance pressures	Learning approach to removing incentives for risk-taking, understanding the perceived pressures contributing to drift, and creating situational awareness to level of associated risk	A patient care tech writes multiple patients vitals on a piece of paper to save time. She documents the wrong vitals under the wrong patient when transcribing the vitals into the electronic medical record
Reckless behavior	Deliberate disregard for risk or consequences associated with the behavior or action	Individuals who choose reckless behavior should be held accountable through disciplinary action	A surgeon refuses to complete the preoperative checklist before proceeding with surgery

over safety and outcomes [7]. Organizations are much better positioned to respond to and fix latent conditions when staff identify and report risks before harm occurs.

Safety Event Reporting: Sounding the Alarm

Understanding how and why errors happen and how systems respond in a learning manner is an important concept when it comes to what to do when something goes wrong. The immediate response to a safety event focuses on containing and stabilizing the situation. When the situation is contained, staff involved should submit a safety event report (SER). SERs are a voluntary means for reporting risks, potential threats, and actual harm events from the viewpoint of those who were directly involved [8]. These reports provide a retrospective account of the event or potential event, contributing factors, and pertinent demographic information. Because those at the sharp end enter SERs, they are often a rich source of information about what could go wrong or why something did go wrong.

Voluntary safety event reporting systems are a widely accepted resource for driving quality and safety improvements [8]. While there are numerous electronic reporting systems for organizations to choose from, they will not be effective without some key considerations. Organizations must consider the following when implementing a reporting system: just culture, usability and access, critical information gathering, and a consistent means for following up on submitted reports [8].

Usability is vital to ensure that SERs are not seen as a burden by staff, and the system collects information necessary to identify risks and drive improvements. In addition to usability, ensuring the appropriate framework for responding to reports in a nonpunitive manner, creating system improvements, and providing feedback to submitters; demonstrates leadership commitment to a systems approach to safety event reporting [8]. SERs are only valuable if people report them, and little can be accomplished if reports are only submitted when something serious happens.

Having a safety event reporting system is not enough if people only use it for major events or when their manager tells them to. Organizations that promote SERs and establish the framework to manage the response end up with a rich database of real and potential system vulnerabilities and the opportunity to fix those vulnerabilitis before they result in harm. These organizations receive more near-miss reports or reports about what could have happened but did not. Developed from Herbert Heinrich's safety triangle, Fig. 4.2, the safety event pyramid, illustrates three main types of safety events: near-misses, precursor events, and serious safety events [9]. Heinrich who spent many years in the insurance industry examining industrial accidents theorized that, for every 1 serious safety event, there are 300 near-miss events and 29 precursor events that signaled risk for harm [9]. Heinrich's theory has been challenged over the years, but the hypothesis remains the same; a serious safety event does not occur without warning, and there are signals within the system that must be identified and acted on to prevent harm.

Near-miss events do not reach the patient but provide signals for system risks that must be addressed. For every serious safety event, numerous near-miss and precursor events signaled weakness in the system, and the failure to address these signals results in a missed opportunity to prevent a serious safety event before it occurs [9].

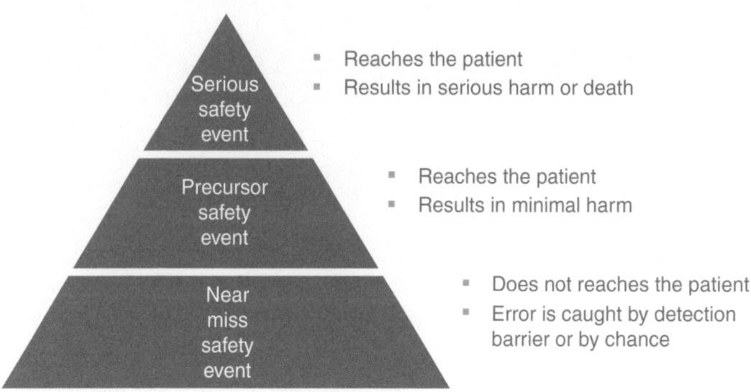

Fig. 4.2 Heinrich's safety event pyramid [9]

Case Study: Hindsight Is 20/20

The nurse notices that the IV pump will not program the correct rate for her medication, despite many attempts to enter the correct numbers. She does not report this because she was able to correct the issue before the error reached the patient.

A few days later, a nurse is programming the IV pump to administer a blood pressure medication. The IV pump administers the medication too quickly and causes the patient to become dizzy. The nurse is certain she programmed the rate correctly, but the IV pump ran much faster than expected. The patient is fine, and the nurse assumes she must have made a mistake setting up the IV pump. She does not report this because there was no lasting patient harm.

A few days later, a nurse is setting up an IV pump to administer a high-risk heart rhythm medication to a critically ill patient. She carefully programs the medication rate into the pump and hits start; time is of the essence for this patient. Within minutes, the patient's heart rhythm becomes erratic, and his heart stops beating. The nurse realizes the medication on the IV pump infused too quickly. She has given this medication hundreds of times and she knows she programmed the pump correctly. The event is classified as a serious safety event, and the nurse submits a safety event report. An analysis of the event reveals an error in the pump software that resulted in the medication infusing too quickly. When this is discussed at grand rounds, several nurses report similar issues with IV pumps.

Imagine if the nurse in the first event reported the unusual response from the IV pump immediately. The software malfunction could have been identified before a serious safety event occurred. Healthcare is risky, and the stakes are high; early identification followed by a systems-focused response is one of the best defenses we have to prevent harm [8].

Tools for Safety

There exists a myriad of tools to mitigate risk and reduce harm. Response to risk is proactive or reactive but requires a thorough and objective review of system vulnerabilities. The following sections highlight a number of relatively simple tools for analyzing error, mitigating risk, and preventing harm.

Tools for Safety: Simple Behaviors to Decrease Harm

Human error is a contributor to all safety events, but application of simple error prevention techniques or behaviors can help people make the right decision in the right situations [10]. Table 4.2

Table 4.2 Solutions for patient safety: error prevention techniques [10]

Error prevention technique	When to use it	Examples
ARCC *A*sk a question Make a *R*equest Voice a *C*oncern *C*hain of command	Use ARCC when you believe there is a situation that threatens the safety of patients or staff. Use this technique to escalate a situation in which your concern is not being addressed	A surgeon is about to begin a procedure without completing a preoperative checklist. The nurse intervenes *A*: "Dr. Smith, are we supposed to complete the checklist before starting?" (Dr. Smith ignores the nurse) *R*: "Dr. Smith, I am requesting that we take a few minutes to complete the checklist before we start." (Dr. Smith says the checklist is wasting his time) *C*: "Dr. Smith, I am concerned about the risk of starting without completing the checklist." (Dr. Smith, picks up his instrument to begin) *C*: "Dr. Smith, before I can help you, I need to speak with my supervisor because the policy states that we complete the checklist first"

(continued)

Table 4.2 (continued)

Error prevention technique	When to use it	Examples
STAR *S*top: Focus on the task *T*hink: What needs to be done *A*ct: Perform the task *R*eview: Evaluate the result	STAR is a quick self-check that helps to prevent skills-based errors that occur when our attention is taken away from a task (distractions, fatigue, time pressures, etc.). STAR can be done quickly before taking action	The doctor is entering a medication order when she is interrupted with a question from a colleague. Before submitting the order, the doctor stops to review the order, thinks through the correct process for ordering, makes any necessary changes to the order, and reviews the order before submitting it
Validate and verify and peer checks	When something does not seem right, it does not make sense, or you have never done it before, validate by assessing the source of the information or the situation and verify (peer check) by asking an expert for an external check of your assessment. Validate and verify before you act It helps to prevent rule-based and knowledge-based errors	A radiologist is looking at X-rays and thinks he might see a broken bone but is not sure. He asks a colleague to review the x-ray, and the colleague confirms that the bone is broken
Closed-loop communication	Repeating back information received to ensure accuracy. Prevents errors related to misinterpreted messages during information exchange	Physician: Give 1 mg of epinephrine IV now Nurse: Repeats back to the physician, I am going to give 1 mg of epinephrine IV now

outlines just a few of the error prevention behaviors recommended by Solutions for Patient Safety, the largest pediatric collaborative for safety in the United States, including when and how to apply these techniques [10]. When teaching these behaviors, it is important to emphasize that the behavior must be used before the individual performs an action to be effective. Error prevention behaviors are widely applicable in healthcare organizations and should be included in the training of all staff regardless of roles.

Tools for Safety: Detecting Errors Before They happen

While much of the response to an error is retrospective, tools are available to address and mitigate risk proactively. The Failure Modes and Effects Analysis (FMEA) analyzes processes to identify where and why the process may fail and the resulting consequences. FMEAs are effective for evaluating new processes, process changes or new applications, and analyzing risk in existing processes [11].

The process outlined below is a basic overview of how to complete an FMEA. Please ensure that you are utilizing the process and resources approved by your organization. The first step of an FMEA is to define the process and assemble a multidisciplinary team of stakeholders to systematically review the process and work through the following steps [11]:

1. Determine the scope of the FMEA: Are we looking at the whole process or just a part of it?
2. Identify the failure modes for each step: What things could go wrong?
3. Determine the consequences (effects) and severity (S) rating: On a scale of 1–10, how bad will it be?
4. Identify the causes of failure and occurrence (O) rating: Why and how often could things go wrong?
5. Identify the defenses in place to prevent failure and detection (D) rating: Are there safeguards in place to prevent or stop the failure, and how will we know?
6. Finally, calculate the risk priority number (RPN) $S \times D \times O = RPN$: How do we know what to fix first?

The RPN is used to prioritize high-risk failure modes and assist the FMEA team in creating a comprehensive action plan. Higher RPNs are generally prioritized first. Action plans should include input from all stakeholders, an owner for each action item, metrics to determine the outcome, and a standardized plan for follow-up. Action items do not reduce risk if they do not happen. Setting a cadence for routine progress check-ins establishes accountability for the completion of action items and a chance to address barriers or challenges to implementation. FMEAs that result in completed action plans are effective tools for mitigating harm before it occurs [11].

Tools for Safety: Retrospective Response to Safety Events

Healthcare is a risky and complicated system. Errors will happen. Despite our best efforts, the majority of those errors are the result of human behaviors or actions [2, 10]. Organizations choose to respond by blaming the person involved or using the event as a learning opportunity to better the system. Apparent cause analyses (ACA) and root cause analyses (RCA) are widely used tools for analyzing events, identifying causes, and creating system improvements.

ACAs and RCAs are distinctly different in many ways. ACAs are primarily utilized for near-miss and precursor events that are limited in scope and result in minimal or no harm [12, 13]. Teams focus on identifying and correcting as many proximate or apparent causes as possible to reduce the likelihood of a repeat event. RCAs are primarily utilized for serious safety events and precursor events where harm reaches the patient. RCAs are resource-intensive, lengthy reviews that identify the most basic causal factor (root cause) and action items to prevent recurrence [13]. The tree below illustrates the difference between apparent and root causes (Fig. 4.3).

The event is just a symptom of the underlying problem, but it is often what we see most clearly (leaves on the tree). Apparent causes are those system causes that may be barely visible just above the ground (base of the tree). Root causes are what feed the entire system (tree) and will result in an error if not corrected. Root causes require significant digging as they are the least visible contributor to safety events. The goal of ACAs and RCAs is not getting distracted by the most obvious signs and looking deeper to find the real cause.

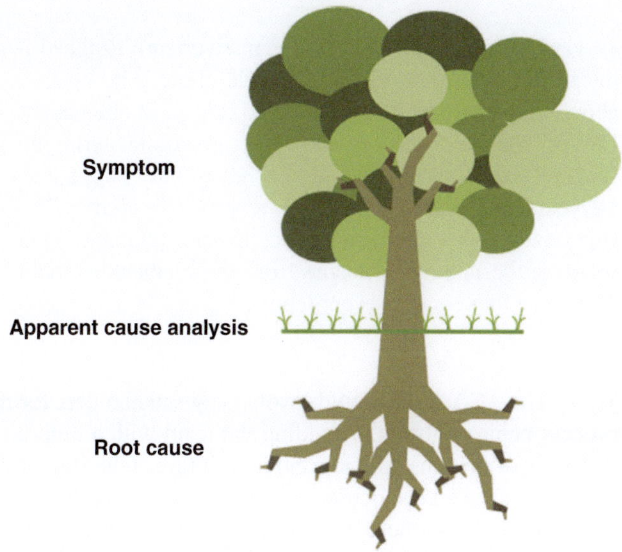

Fig. 4.3 Apparent versus root causes

Tools for Safety: Looking for the Apparent Causes

This section focuses on the ACA process. RCAs should be completed by a trained facilitator with a strong knowledge of safety science and systems thinking. Please utilize the resources and tools approved by your organization when completing a cause analysis. Below are the key elements to consider when initiating an ACA [13].

- *Facilitator*: Cause analyses facilitators need strong facilitation skills and a basic understanding of safety science and systems thinking. The facilitator keeps the team focused on the system, manages expectations, and helps the team move through systematic analysis and action plan [13].
- *Event*: ACAs are most successful for events that involve or impact <4 departments, deviate from an established process, have a clear timeline, and are limited in scope to allow the analysis to be done in 90 minutes to 2 hours [13].

The adult form of a vaccine is inadvertently stocked in the medication room of the pediatric clinic. The nurse is about to administer the vaccine to a 5-year-old patient. Using STAR to check her actions before administering the vaccine, she notices that the vial says "Use for patients 18 years and older." The nurse reports the event to her supervisor, who immediately calls the pharmacy and removes the incorrect vaccine from the medication room. The nurse files a safety event report.

- *Team*: The ACA team should involve key stakeholders for the process being analyzed. Providing the team with a high-level overview of systems thinking and just culture at the start of the ACA keeps the teams focused on latent conditions [13]. Front-line expertise from those who know the work best is beneficial to identifying the difference between how we believe the work is being done versus how work is really being done i.e., work-arounds or drift.

The pediatric clinic team decides to do an ACA on the vaccine event. They ask pharmacy to be part of the team because they are involved in stocking the medication.

- *Analysis*: Using an analysis tool guides the team in reviewing the sequence of events and identifying the apparent causes and prevents focusing on active failures [13]. The five "whys" is a commonly used and easily applied tool for looking beneath the actions of an individual, understanding why these actions made sense at the moment, and what about the system supported these actions at the moment [13]. The apparent causes are the gaps in the system that failed to identify or prevent the error from occurring.

The team reviews the event step by step. They compare the vaccine stocking process as it should have happened with how the process did happen in this event. The team uses the five "whys" to find the apparent causes.

- How did this happen? The pharmacy tech chose the wrong vaccine to stock.
- Why? She got distracted by a phone call while stocking and grabbed the wrong vial.
- Why? Because the pediatric and adult vials are identical and she did not realize it was the wrong vial.
- Why? Because the techs do not scan the vaccines when stocking.

The team realized that the techs were not scanning the vaccine while stocking, so there was no hard stop of safeguard in place other than double-checks by humans (the tech was distracted in this case) to prevent this error from happening.

- *Action plan*: If the action items do not address the causes, the ACA will not be successful. The facilitator should guide the team towards highly reliable actions that focus on system improvements [12, 13]. Reliable action items focus on creating processes and systems (forcing functions, standardization, physical plant changes) to mitigate error as opposed to relying on people (education, warning signs) to prevent harm [12, 13].

The pharmacy team members chose to update the scanners in the medication room to include vaccines and educate the pharmacy techs about how to use the scanners. The pharmacy team members will audit the scanning log during the implementation period to ensure the new process is being followed and address any issues that arise. The nursing team will also scan the vaccine prior to administration to ensure multiple layers of safeguards in the system.

- *Follow-up*: Establishing a process for follow-up on action items creates accountability for completion and allows the team to address barriers to implementation [13]. Follow-up can be in the form of a brief meeting or phone call for stakeholders to review progress. ACAs will not achieve the desired outcome if the action items are not completed.

Three months after initiating the scanning process in the pediatric clinic, the pharmacy and nursing teams meet to discuss progress. Vaccine scanning during stocking is at 90%, but the techs report that it takes them 10 minutes longer to complete stocking. The pharmacy team is adjusting the tech's stocking schedule to accommodate this. The nursing team also reports 90% compliance with scanning and is working with the frontline staff to address any barriers.

Thorough analysis and strong action plans significantly contribute to reducing the likelihood of recurrence [12, 13]. Don't get distracted by the leaves on the tree, and follow a systematic approach for digging down to the apparent causes to drive sustainable and successful system improvement. There are numerous resources available to help you learn basic safety science, systems thinking, and facilitation skills. Your organization likely has a safety officer or staff member who is proficient in these skills and able to guide you through the process approved by your system.

Error: Closing the Loop

Healthcare may be risky, and people are prone to error, but relatively simple tools and techniques exist to reduce vulnerability and create lasting system improvements. Errors and safety events are learning experiences, and organizations should respond by creating safer systems to safeguard the people at the sharp end of care and the patients they care for. Moving focus from human error to system error shifts the paradigm from reactive to proactive and allows organizations to get in front of risks before harm occurs.

References

1. Kohn LT, Corrigan JM. To err is human: building a safer health system. Washington, DC: National Academies Press; 2000.
2. Reason J. Human error: models and management. Wes J Med [Internet]. 2000 [cited 2020 July 1];176(6):393–6. Available from: https://www.ncbi.nlm.nih.gov/pmc/articles/PMC1117770/. https://doi.org/10.1136/ewjm.172.6.393.
3. Altabbakh H, Murray SL. Applying the Swiss Cheese model of accident causation. In: Annual international conference of the American Society for Engineering Management: 2011 October 19–22. Lubbock, TX: American Society for Engineering Management; 2011. p. 301–7.
4. Paine LA. Safe and just culture. In: Annual quality conference: 2015 March 18. Louisville: Kentucky Hospital Association; [cited 2020 June 26]. Available from: http://www.kipsq.org/Portals/26/Documents/KIPSQJustCulture.pdf
5. Amalberti R, et al. Violations and migrations in health care: a framework for understanding and management. Qual Saf Health Care [internet]. 2006 [cited 2020, July 30];15:66–71. Available from: https://www.ncbi.nlm.nih.gov/pmc/articles/PMC2464877/. https://doi.org/10.1136/qshc.2005.015982.
6. North Carolina Board of Nursing. What could happen: the consequences of "practice drift"…is it worth the risk? [Course bulletin on the internet]. Fall; 2016 [cited 1 July 2020]. 7p. Available from: https://www.ncbon.com/vdownloads/course-bulletin-offerings-articles/bulletin-article-fall-2016-practice-drift.pdf
7. Frankel AS, et al. Fair and just culture, team behavior, and leadership engagement: the tools to achieve high reliability. Health Serv Res [Internet]. 2006 [cited 2020 July 1];41(4 Part 2):690–709. Available from: https://www.semanticscholar.org/paper/Fair-and-just-culture%2C-team-behavior%2C-and-The-tools-Frankel-Leonard/a19e684be606dd4425b838f876d4852ad1b562d6. https://doi.org/10.1111/j.1475-6773.2006.00572.x.
8. Patient Safety Primer: Reporting Patient Safety Events. Agency for healthcare research and quality. 2019 [cited 28, June 2020]. Available at: https://psnet.ahrq.gov/primer/reporting-patient-safety-events

9. Yorio PL, Moore SM. Examining factors that influence the existence of Heinrich's safety triangle using site-specific H&S data from more than 25,000 establishments. Risk Anal [Internet]. 2017 [cited 29 June 2020];38(4):839–52. Available from: https://pubmed.ncbi.nlm.nih.gov/28768045/. https://doi.org/10.1111/risa.12869.
10. Creating a culture of safety and high reliability at Children's Hospital's Solutions for Patient Safety Network Hospitals handbook: behavior expectations for safety and performance excellence [Internet]. Solutions for patient safety. 2018 [cited 28 June 2020], p 37. Available at: https://portal.solutionsforpatientsafety.org/CulturalDomains/hrerrorprevention/_layouts/15/WopiFrame2.aspx?sourcedoc=%7B60CB4994-0DAF-41C3-BD4A-E8D465939594%7D&file=EP_Handbook_SPS.docx&action=default&CT=1593631835052&OR=DocLibClassicUI&AuthResend1908BC2350124b5095AB75012FA405BA
11. Failure Modes and Effects Analysis (FMEA) [Internet]. 2020 [Cited 29 June 2020]. Available at: https://asq.org/quality-resources/fmea
12. Crandall K, et al. Improving apparent cause analysis reliability: a quality improvement initiative. Pediatr Qual Saf [Internet]. 2017 [cited 26 June 2020];v2(3). Available at: https://www.semanticscholar.org/paper/Improving-Apparent-Cause-Analysis-Reliability%3A-A-Crandall-Sten/748f8baff4b2ef5cc7ca18f3799912a93ecca9fa. https://doi.org/10.1097/pq9.000000000000002.
13. Parikh K, et al. Apparent cause analysis: a safety tool. Pediatrics [Internet]. 2020 [cited 27 June 2020];145(5). Available at: https://doi.org/10.1542/peds.2019-1819.

5 Employee and Staff Safety

Janice J. Mason and Alia Fink

Why Employee and Staff Safety?

In nursing school, in the early 1990s and early 2000s, there was a lot of focus on patient safety and not much focus on employee safety in healthcare settings. During this time, it was very common during clinical learning shifts at local hospitals to observe nurses, technicians, respiratory therapists, environmental services workers, and physicians working long hours with few breaks. The patients were large, often immobile, and sometimes violent toward staff. When nurses were asked about these tough conditions, they often shrugged and talked about ways they coped with the physical and emotional demands. Many nurses talked about injuries and illnesses acquired at work. An observer can quickly get the sense that the staff accepted risky conditions and workplace injuries as a normal part of working in healthcare. Adapting to the status quo is often contagious. To maintain good health and

J. J. Mason (✉)
Department of Nursing Science, Professional Practice & Quality, Children's National Hospital, Washington, DC, USA
e-mail: jmason@childrensnational.org

A. Fink
Performance Improvement Department, Children's National Hospital, Washington, DC, USA
e-mail: afink@childrensnational.org

R. Roberts-Turner, R. K. Shah (eds.), *Pocket Guide to Quality Improvement in Healthcare*,
https://doi.org/10.1007/978-3-030-70780-4_5

minimize risks, staff took care of themselves through good self-care practices. But as we know, bubble baths, chocolate, and even the best mindfulness meditation practice aren't enough to create and maintain a safe healthcare workplace for all.

Safety in the workplace is paramount, and every employer and employee must make safety a number one priority to establish a safe and healthy work environment. Safety in the workplace can refer to both physical and psychological safety. In both instances, it means having a workplace that's reasonably free from danger to all employees and actively preventing the workplace from becoming unsafe. As hospital nursing leaders with a combined experience of over 45 years, we believe that a safe workplace in healthcare is one where employees are able to perform at their best and where systems and processes are set up to support employees' health and well-being and are continuously improved and adapted based on organizational and environmental changes. The first step is actually eliminating harm in the workplace. We argue that using quality improvement methods is an effective way to reduce and eliminate harm. Thus, employee safety and quality improvement are inherently intertwined.

Nothing illustrates this point better than when Paul O'Neil became CEO of Alcoa, the Aluminum Company of America, in 1987. As he began his tenure, he announced that worker safety would be the company's priority. O'Neil made it clear that he intended to get to zero worker injuries. This radical idea was first met with shock and skepticism. However, once O'Neil prioritized workplace safety, over the next 13 years, Alcoa's profits soared. O'Neil made workplace safety a keystone habit, one that when changed facilitates improvements in other systems and processes in the workplace [1].

In an effort to improve the work environment, employee safety became top of mind at our large urban pediatric academic medical center with a staff of 7,000 employees. As other hospitals were beginning to explore improving employee safety and its relationship with patient safety, our chief executive officer and board asked us to do the same. Leadership looked closely at its employee injury rate and found that it was higher than other pediatric hospitals. At the urging and leadership of our chief executive officer, in 2017, the hospital decided to embark on a journey to improve workplace safety. Using quality improvement methods, we improved employee safety at our hospital over a 3-year period. Serious injuries, those that required staff to miss work or be reassigned, decreased by 37%.

Structure, Process, and Outcomes

The foundational Donabedian concepts of structure and process leading to desired outcomes in quality improvement also apply to an effective employee safety program [2]. At our pediatric academic medical center, a structure was set up to include a committee of leaders, representing many different areas from the organization who had a stake in employee safety. Leaders from nursing, occupational health, environmental services, security, safety and quality, workers' compensation, infection control, and several other departments came together to work on this issue. Each representative led a team of staff from their areas who worked on the processes they determined would improve staff safety. Just like in quality improvement projects, when the structure and processes are strong, the outcomes follow. Teams that are representative of the workforce help ease the change necessary for improvement.

With change comes anxiety and often resistance. Though change is constant, humans crave predictability and routine. We've heard nurses say many times that a practice or process is done in healthcare "because that's how we've always done it." Clinging to tradition may soothe anxious workers, but it does not help advance quality or safety in the workplace.

A safe workplace depends on the collaboration between employers and employees. A primary responsibility of an employer is to provide a safe and productive work environment for employees. Regardless of the type of work employees perform, they should never be in a position where their physical safety is in jeopardy. Employers have an obligation to protect employees from injury and illness on the job. Protecting employees from accidents and injuries in the workplace can decrease expenses to the organization. For example, a reduction in workplace injuries and illnesses likely reduces workers' compensation claims and lost workdays.

The sole responsibility of maintaining a safe work environment not only lies with employers, the entire workforce must recognize that employee safety and health is essential to the mission and significant to the financial viability of the workplace. Employees need to assess the condition of the work environment and take the necessary precautions while performing their duties; for example, prior to handling equipment and hazardous substances that might pose a safety risk, employees should complete the necessary education and training to reduce harm and injuries. Employees should immediately report any identified hazards to management. To avoid fatigue, stress, and burnout, which are contributors to workplace accidents, employees should take scheduled breaks.

At our pediatric academic medical center, the employee safety program was intended to be a large organization-wide project; the hospital's leadership commissioned a steering committee to oversee the subcommittees who would perform the analysis and intervention implementation. The project was divided into five subcommittees: overexertion; sharps; blood and body fluids; verbal and physical violence; slips, trips, and falls. Specific stakeholders from each area comprised the leadership and membership in each subcommittee. Each subcommittee used the same quality improvement methods, primarily, the Institute for Healthcare Improvement's Model for Improvement, to execute their project [3]. They all focused on establishing strong structures and processes. They created key drivers, conducted literature reviews, and researched best practices from industry experts. They used Plan-Do-Study-Act cycles to test interventions and then scale them up. As expected, despite using the same methods, each subcommittee has a unique improvement story.

Overexertion Injuries and Safe Patient Handling

Alan's Story

Alan*, a seasoned nurse, was taking care of a very ill 18-year-old girl in an intensive care unit who could not move on her own. She was a large patient, and when he was turning her in bed, he felt a pop in his back. Unable to move because of excruciating pain, he went to the nearest emergency department. He ended up needing back surgery for a disk injury.

At home and out of work for many months experiencing back pain, Alan became depressed. He had a hard time weaning off of his opioid pain pills after surgery. In addition to the chronic pain, he was constantly worried about his lost income and not being able to support his family. His family encouraged him to seek mental health support and suggested addiction treatment. At first, he was resistant to ask for help. He couldn't understand how in 1 day he went from being a healthy, active, 48-year-old nurse to being unable to provide for his family, depressed, and dependent on pain pills.

Two months after his injury, his wife and best friend sat down with him for an intervention. They convinced him to get help for his depression and pain pill use. With mental health support, addiction treatment, and physical therapy, Alan slowly began to feel better. He still had chronic back pain but was able to wean off the opioids. He worked hard to develop other coping strategies and regain some of his self-confidence. He was lucky that his family and friends supported him through his difficult journey. When Alan finally returned to work, he had a lift restriction that prevented him from doing any manual lifting of patients. Alan began to tell his story to colleagues, to encourage them to use lift equipment to move patients instead of moving them manually. In situations where lift equipment is not available, Alan urged his colleagues to ask for assistance to avoid injury to themselves and the patient.

According to the National Safety Council, overexertion injuries are caused by [4]:

- Directing excessive physical effort at an object (lifting, pulling, carrying, throwing)
- Repetitive motion (typing, using tools or instruments)
- Free bodily motion (bending, crawling, twisting, kneeling)

Overexertion is a leading cause of injury for all age groups. In 2014, hospitals treated 3,132,271 overexertion-related injuries [6]. Industries are impacted financially from employees that experienced overexertion injuries. For example, the consequences of work-related musculoskeletal injuries among healthcare employees are substantial, along with higher employer costs due to medical expenses, disability compensation, and litigation [4–7].

Overexertion causes 35% of all work-related injuries and is the #1 reason for lost workdays. By far, it is the largest contributor to workers' compensation costs, more than $15 billion or 25% of the total cost in 2012, according to Injury Facts 2016®. More than 322,000 people missed work that year due to overexertion. In 2014, there were 68,720 work-related injuries in the health services and education industry [6].

The types of movements that can lead to strains and sprains (the most often reported nature of injuries) often seem harmless, but excessive physical efforts account for nearly half of overexertion injuries occurring in the trunk of the body, primarily the back. Another large portion occurs in the shoulder. These injuries often result from a single, intensive use of force while trying to lift, pull, or throw an object.

Safe Lifting

In the workplace, musculoskeletal injuries from lifting and moving patients are common. Using unsafe or careless lifting techniques can put employees at risk for a serious back injury. Proper safe lifting techniques are recommended to avoid injuries [6].

Basic best practices for lifting:

- Stabilize your body by keeping your feet shoulder-width apart.
- Squat and let your leg muscles do the heavy lifting.

- Avoid bending and relying on your back muscles.
- Avoid twisting while lifting.
- Seek assistance when lifting heavy patients or equipment.
- When possible, use safe lift assistive devices or equipment for heavy lifts.

These best practices work well for lifting and moving objects, but lifting and moving people is quite different. It is a myth that using proper body mechanics alone will prevent an overexertion injury when lifting or moving patients [5]. Safe patient handling and movement programs are helpful to prevent risk of injury to patients and healthcare workers. Rather than using people to lift, move, reposition, or transfer patients, it is recommended that healthcare facilities provide and train employees on the proper use of safe patient handling equipment to decrease injuries. Implementing safe patient handling practices will also reduce a healthcare facility's financial burden with regard to patient claims and workers' compensation claims [7].

Safe patient handling and movement programs can help prevent what happened to Alan from happening to other healthcare workers. The foundation of a safe patient handling and movement program is a clear policy and procedure detailing when and how to use assistive equipment like mechanical patient lifts and friction reducing slider sheets.

Making the change to using equipment to assist with lifting and moving patients can be a difficult transition for healthcare staff if they have been manually lifting and moving patients for a long time. Many myths exist in healthcare about patient lifting. Some of these myths are that using equipment to lift patients takes more time and is less safe for patients. In fact, safe patient handling practices and equipment actually save time and are safer for patients than manual lifting. Both formal and informal leadership are necessary for safe patient handling practice changes to occur successfully. Formal leaders can advocate for and purchase safe patient handling equipment and can support and guide staff in using it. Informal leaders can readily support the change and influence their peers, by sharing their confidence in using equipment to safely move patients.

When the culture in an organization changes and staff consistently use safe patient handling equipment to move patients, employee overexertion injuries decrease. Attention to general workplace ergonomics is also important for preventing overexertion injuries.

Sharps and Blood and Body Fluids

Carol's Story

Carol*, a surgical fellow, was performing an appendectomy on a 9-year-old boy. Carol was nearing the end of a long shift after a stretch of several back-to-back days working at the hospital. Carol had not slept much the night before because she was on call. The appendectomy surgery had gone smoothly, and Carol was suturing the wound closed. She was humming along as she sutured, when suddenly she felt a sharp stick through her glove in her finger. The curved suture needle stuck her. She froze and told the team what just happened. The other surgeon present took over, and Carol left to wash her finger and report the injury. Both Carol and the patient had to undergo testing for blood-borne pathogens, and Carol had to take prophylactic medications until she found out if she had contracted any infections. The experience was incredibly stressful for Carol, her family, and the operating room staff.

Sharps and needlestick injuries are injuries to the skin that are caused by sharp instruments and hollow-bore needles (lancet, scalpels, glass, hypodermic needles, butterfly needles, suture needles, syringe needles, IV catheter stylets) that accidentally penetrate the skin in a healthcare setting [8–10].

According to the Centers for Disease Control and Prevention (CDC), the most common causes that are related to sharps and needlestick injuries include but are not limited to [8, 13]:

- Recapping needles after use
- Failure to use sharps container to dispose needles after use
- Lack of sharps disposal containers

- Overfilled sharps disposal containers
- Lack of safety needles and safety devices
- Passing of sharp instruments from hand to hand in the operating room
- Patient movement during procedures
- Lack of staff education, training, and awareness
- Underreporting of sharps and needlestick injuries

Most exposure to sharps and needlestick injuries are known to occur in the patient's room, the emergency department, and the operating room [14]. As a result of a lack of surveillance and underreporting of sharps and needlestick injuries, incidence rates and national benchmarked data are insufficient and difficult to obtain [12]. Sharps and needlestick injuries are underreported by 58–90% [18, 19]. Several reasons why sharps and needlestick injuries are underreported are due to "time constraints, perception that the percutaneous injury does not represent a significant exposure, lack of knowledge about the reporting mechanism and concern about confidentiality and professional discrimination" [17].

Health concerns including patient's blood and body fluid (BBF) exposures to healthcare workers from sharps and needlestick injuries can cause infectious diseases, such as human immunodeficiency virus (HIV), hepatitis B virus (HBV), and hepatitis C virus (HCV) [9, 16]. If healthcare workers become infected and are not treated, they can develop serious acute and chronic diseases that can potentially lead to death [9, 17].

Sharps and needlestick injuries can have a financial impact to the healthcare organization and to the healthcare worker. Medical treatments, missed time at work, work productivity, workman's compensation payouts, and litigations are financial consequences that can occur as a result of sharps and needlestick injuries in the workplace [14].

A complete approach using a blend of various strategies should be used to reduce sharps and needlestick injuries to avoid blood and body fluid exposures. Preventative strategies include [16–20]:

- Use of safety needles/devices and needleless connectors
- Reduce recapping of needles
- Proper patient holding technique
- Availability of sharps disposal container
- Immediate disposal of sharps and needles after use
- Frequent emptying of sharps disposal container to reduce overfill
- Eliminate unnecessary injections
- Increase reporting of sharps and needlestick injuries
- Frequent staff education, training, and awareness

A multidisciplinary team with physicians and surgeons, nurses, ancillary staff, infection control, and materials management is necessary to make a lasting impact on sharps injuries and blood and body fluid exposures. Since these types of injuries occur during patient care or surgical procedures, tackling both problems with one team can be effective in driving improvement.

Interventions that can prevent injuries and exposures like Carol's from happening again include programs to reduce fatigue and to reinforce standardized sharps handling guidelines. Purchasing needleless devices to replace needles, whenever possible, and making needleless equipment like blood transfer devices, needleless connectors, and vial access devices accessible and available to staff are also effective interventions.

Blood and body fluid exposures occur when a patient's blood or body fluids come into contact with a healthcare provider's skin or mucous membranes, such as the eyes, nose, or mouth. Employees are at risk for the same communicable diseases, like hepatitis and HIV, from these exposures as they are from sharps injuries. The best way to prevent a patient's blood or body fluids from coming into contact with an employee's skin or mucous membranes is to use personal protective equipment (PPE), like gowns, gloves, masks, and face shields, properly and consistently when performing any procedure at risk for a fluid exposure.

Increasing availability of PPE close to the point of care and auditing staff compliance of properly wearing PPE can be effective strategies to prevent blood and body fluid exposures. Employees need regular feedback on their PPE compliance, as well as ongoing training and reinforcement of correct PPE usage.

Sharps injuries and blood and body fluid exposures are preventable. With a quality improvement and multidisciplinary team approach, organizations can be successful in reducing these injuries and the impact they have on staff and patients.

Slips, Trips, and Falls

Marcia's Story

Marcia* is an emergency department physician with 20 years of experience. As she entered the building on a rainy day one October, she slipped and fell on the slick floor of the entryway and landed on her tailbone. She got up slowly with help from other employees. She was a bit embarrassed, as she had prided herself on maintaining her fitness. Her tailbone felt quite painful, and she realized she should get an x-ray and get examined by a doctor. She was diagnosed with a small tailbone fracture from her fall and needed to miss a substantial amount of work. It took 12 weeks for her tailbone fracture to heal.

In terms of severity, slips, trips, and falls (37%) are leading causes of workplace injuries [21, 22]. The most common hazards that lead to workplace falls in healthcare include spills, trip hazards, weather conditions, inadequate lighting, and problems with stairs and stair rails. Slips and trips can lead to strains and sprain injuries to the shoulders, back, and neck. A slip is caused by a loss of friction between your footwear and the floor, and a trip is caused by a physical obstacle like a loose tile, objects in a walk path, cracked sidewalk, or floor surface that prevents an individual from completing a step [21].

For healthcare and other industries, fall injuries create a considerable financial burden: workers' compensation and medical costs associated with occupational fall incidents have been estimated at $70 billion annually in the United Sates [22].

Occupational slips, trips, and falls are preventable. Evidence suggests that facility-wide programs targeting common slip, trip, and fall hazards can reduce a facility's injury rate. Wet floor signs should be used when floors are slippery and wet, spills should be cleaned up immediately, and during the winter fast removal of ice and snow from walkways and sidewalks [23].

Tips to prevent falls from slips [21, 23]:

- Inspect floor surfaces often and clean up hazards.
- Place warning signs in damp or wet areas.
- Maintain good lighting in dark areas.
- Wear proper footwear for the environment.
- Take extra care during icy or snowy weather.

Tips to prevent falls from trips [21, 23]:

- Keep walkways clear of hazards.
- Maintain good lighting in dark areas.
- Pay attention and avoid texting while walking.
- Repair significant cracks and gaps in concrete.
- Inspect work areas for loose cords and cables.
- Keep your path of vision clear when carrying items.
- Use handrails on stairs.

A multidisciplinary team for falls should include diverse stakeholders, like environmental services supervisors and frontline workers, facilities staff, safety personnel, security staff, and regulatory/accreditation representatives. Analyzing the causes of falls in an organization can help determine where to concentrate improvement efforts. For example, if wet floor transitions are the most frequent cause of falls, then targeting interventions to address wet floors would be a good strategy.

Effective interventions to prevent falls from wet floor transitions include deploying long walk-off mats and plastic umbrella bags placed in entrances when it is raining. Pop-up wet floor signs are great because they are stored in tubes on the wall, are easily accessible, and can be used by anyone. Installation of pop-up wet floor signs, along busy hallways and outside of elevators, helps make it easy for staff or visitors to prevent a fall immediately after noticing a wet floor.

Environmental services or facilities leaders need to consistently round in the hospital and parking areas anticipating slips, trips, and falls risks. Equipment in crowded hallways, loose cords in office areas, and dimly lit parking lots are potential injury hazards that should be remedied.

Slips, trips, and falls are preventable in the healthcare environment. With a multidisciplinary team structure, processes and interventions that address the biggest causes of falls in an organization, slips, trips, and falls among healthcare workers can be drastically reduced.

Verbal and Physical Violence

Robert's Story

A teenage patient with a history of behavioral health issues and substance use was admitted to the emergency department with agitation and disorientation. There were multiple caregivers involved in de-escalating the patient and caring for him. Despite the team's best efforts at de-escalation, the patient continued to escalate and required restraint by security and other staff. In the process of restraint, the patient hit Robert*, one of the security officers, knocking him backward off of his feet. He lost consciousness, sustained a closed head injury, and needed 10 months of intensive medical treatment before being able to return to work. The injury was devastating for Robert, his family, and the department. Robert's story demonstrates the challenge of caring for patients with violent behaviors while keeping staff safe. Healthcare workers come to work, wanting to help their patients and families. The impact of fear of getting hurt at work and of injuries from violent patients and families is profound.

Workplace violence, described as any physical assault, verbal abuse, or threatening disruptive behavior in the workplace, can occur anywhere, but certain industries such as healthcare are prone to increase physical and verbal violence from patients, visitors, and employees [24]. In 2018, workplace assaults resulted in 20,790 injuries and illnesses involving days away from work and 453 fatalities [25].

Ways in which organizations can address workplace violence include [24, 26]:

- Employee training and creating an emergency action plan
- Conducting mock training exercises with local law enforcement
- Adopting a zero-tolerance policy toward workplace violence
- Creating a system that allows employees to report violent activities
- Reporting unusual employee behavior to human resources
- Implementing enforcement procedures to protect employees
- Identifying appropriate resources to support injured healthcare workers

Perhaps the most complex and challenging of all the employee safety areas is violence prevention in the hospital and healthcare environment. Most hospitals struggle with this challenge and are working to reduce violence in the workplace. Patients with behavioral health issues can unfortunately escalate and harm themselves or their caregivers. They do not have a moral problem; rather, their illnesses can increase their volatility. People with behavioral health challenges deserve compassionate and specialized care while maintaining a safe environment for everyone involved. Stress of the healthcare environment itself can trigger violent behaviors in staff, patients, and families. Parents of hospitalized children can quickly become overwhelmed and do not always have robust support systems. At times mounting family frustrations and stressors can facilitate verbal or physical violence toward hospital staff or other family members.

Patients often cause about 70% of violent events toward staff. Parents, visitors, and caregivers cause about 30% of violent events. Parents and caregivers tend to cause the majority of verbal violence incidents, and patients cause the majority of physical violence incidents. Strategies that work to prevent violence from both patients and their families are imperative to keep the hospital environment safe.

An interprofessional team approach to prevent violence toward employees is essential due to the complexity of the problem. Teams should include hospital leadership, security, nurses, psychiatry representatives, physicians, and social workers. Analysis of violent events can help lead the team to target the highest risk areas in the hospital, likely the emergency department, psychiatry units if there are such areas, or other specific areas that care for patients with behavioral health problems.

Finding the right combination of tools to reduce workplace violence is difficult and unique to each healthcare setting. Crisis prevention programs that train staff in physical and verbal de-escalation can be very effective in preventing violence, as verbal violence can escalate to physical violence. Personal protective equipment like cut-resistant sleeves work to prevent bites, scratches, and cuts can be worn as part of a healthcare worker's uniform. Using simulations and tabletop response drills for staff to practice responding to patients in behavioral health crises can help prepare staff to respond to violent situations.

Ultimately, healthcare organizations need to invest in enough resources and support for staff to prevent and manage violent situations in the workplace.

Conclusion

Quality improvement and employee and staff safety are inherently intertwined. Employees need a safe work environment in order to do their jobs efficiently and effectively. Like patient safety, when employee safety is emphasized, it fosters a collective and continuous commitment by employers and employees in the workplace. Employee safety serves as a foundation for a culture of safety and a culture of continuous quality improvement. Our hospital created a centralized Employee and staff safety program, using quality improvement methodologies that led to measurable improvements in several key areas.

From the beginning, the Employee and Staff Safety Steering Committee realized that in order to successfully strengthen employee safety as a quality improvement initiative, we needed to have a holistic end-to-end view, and it must be at the top of leadership's agenda. Our success was aided by establishing a structure with the right stakeholders in the form of a steering committee and subcommittees.

Executive leadership support and commitment to employee safety, along with interprofessional partnerships, were essential to the success of these initiatives. Leveraging the use of safe devices, safe techniques, safe equipment, and resources has helped to decrease employee injury and harm, and has increased awareness ultimately resulting in a positive shift in our healthcare system's culture of safety.

*Names of injured employee have been changed to protect the privacy of the individuals. However, the employee injury stories included in this chapter are based on real events.

References

1. Duhigg C. The power of habit: why we do what we do in life and business. New York: Random House; 2012.
2. Ayanian JZ, Markel H. Donabedian's lasting framework for health care quality. N Engl J Med. 2016;375(3):205. https://doi.org/10.1056/NEJMp1605101.
3. Institute for Healthcare Improvement. Improving heath and healthcare worldwide [Internet]. 2020 [updated 2020; cited 2020 Jun 6]. Available from: http://www.ihi.org/
4. National Safety Council. Ergonomics-overexertion [Internet]. 2020 [cited 2020 Jun 6]. Available from: https://www.nsc.org/work-safety/safety-topics/ergonomics-overexertion
5. Safe patient handling: busting the myths [Internet]. 2020 [cited 2020 Jun 6]. Available from: https://www.osha.gov/dsg/hospitals/documents/3.1_Mythbusters_508.pdf
6. National Safety Council. Injury facts: the source for injury stats [Internet]. 2020 [cited 2020 Jun 6]. Available from: https://www.nsc.org/membership/member-resources/injury-facts
7. Occupational Safety and Health Administration. Safe patient handling [Internet]. 2020 [cited 2020 Jun 6]. Available from: https://www.osha.gov

8. Centers for Disease Control and Prevention. Workbook for designing, implementing evaluating a sharps injury prevention program [Internet]. 2008 [updated 2015; cited 2020 Jun 6]. Available from: https://www.cdc.gov/sharpssafety/pdf/sharpsworkbook_2008.pdf
9. Riddell A, Kennedy I, Tong CY. Management of sharps injuries in the healthcare setting. BMJ. 2015;351:h3733. https://doi.org/10.1136/bmj.h3733.
10. Wicker S, Stirn AV, Rabenau HF, von Gierke L, Wutzler S, Stephan C. Needlestick injuries: causes, preventability and psychological impact. Infection. 2014;42(3):549–52.
11. Yang L, Mullan B. Reducing needle stick injuries in healthcare occupations: an integrative review of the literature. ISRN Nurs. 2011;2011:315432. https://doi.org/10.5402/2011/315432.
12. Rapiti E, Prüss-Üstün A, Hutin Y. Sharps injuries – assessing the burden of disease from sharps injuries to health-care workers at national and local levels, Environmental burden of disease series, no. 11. Geneva: WHO; 2005.
13. National Institute for Occupational Safety and Health. NIOSH Alert: Preventing needlestick injuries in health care settings. Centers for Disease Control and Prevention. (NIOSH). 2004. United States Department of Health and Human Services. Available from: https://www.cdc.gov/niosh/docs/2000-108/default.html.
14. Perry J, Jagger J. Healthcare worker blood exposure risk: correcting some outdated statistics. Adv Expo Prev. 2003;6(3):28–3.
15. Lavoie MC, Verbeek JH, Pahwa M. Devices for preventing percutaneous exposure injuries caused by needles in healthcare personnel. Cochrane Database Syst Rev. 2014;3:CD0097401.
16. Higginson R, Parry A. Needlestick injuries and safety syringes: a review of the literature. Br J Nurs. 2013;22(8):S4, S6–8, S10
17. Hadaway L. Needlestick injuries, short peripheral catheters, and health care worker risks. J Infus Nurs. 2012;35(3):164–78.
18. Alvarado F, Panlilio A, Cardo D, NaSH Surveillance Group. Percutaneous injury reporting in U.S. hospitals, 1998. In: Program and abstracts of the 4th decennial international conference on nosocomial and healthcare-associated infections. Atlanta: Centers for Disease Control and Prevention. Abstract P-S2–38. Trim JC, Elliott TSJ. A review of sharp injuries and preventative strategies. J Hosp Infect. 2003;53:237–42. Available from: www.ncbi.nlm.nih.gov/pubmed/12660120.
19. Trim JC, Adams D, Elliott TS. Healthcare workers' knowledge of inoculation injuries and glove use. Br J Nurs. 2003;12(4):215–21.
20. De Carli G, Abiteboul D, Puro V. The importance of implementing safe sharps practices in the laboratory setting in Europe. Biochem Med (Zagreb). 2014;24(1):45–56.

21. Baratta R. Trip vs. slip: a biomechanic view [Internet]. 2012 [cited 2020 Jun10]. Available from: https://www.claimsjournal.com/magazines/idea-exchange/2012/01/30/200756.htm
22. NSC. Report on injuries in America 2002. Itasca, IL: National Safety Council 2020. Available from: https://www.nsc.org/membership/member-resources/injury-facts.
23. Bell JL, Collins JW, Tiesman HM, et al. Slip, trip, and fall injuries among nursing care facility workers. Workplace Health Saf. 2013;61(4):147–52. https://doi.org/10.1177/216507991306100402.
24. National Safety Council. Assaults fourth leading cause of workplace death [Internet]. 2020 [cited 2020 Jun 14]. Available from: https://www.nsc.org/work-safety/safety-topics/workplace-violence
25. National Safety Council. Injury facts: assault at work [Internet]. 2020 [cited 2020 Jun 14]. Available from: https://injuryfacts.nsc.org/work/safety-topics/assault/
26. Occupational Safety and Health Administration. Workplace violence [Internet]. 2020 [cited 2020 Jun 20]. Available from: www.osha.gov

6 Regulatory and Accreditation

Layla San Martin

Introduction

In all my years in healthcare, I will never forget the first time I was at work in the cardiac intensive care unit and overheard an announcement: "The Joint Commission is here for our triennial survey, please prepare your areas!" As a cold sweat drew upon my brow, pins and needles shot up my spine, a sinking pit grew in my stomach, and I had NO IDEA what was happening! Staff began to scramble, drinks and snacks put away, hallways cleared of any unused chairs and bedside tables, and supplies found a home (for the first time in weeks). Logs were checked, charts (paper back in the day) were quickly completed, and the nurse's station was empty!

This was my first experience with a regulatory survey, and it seemed like a big deal! As the surveyors walked around the unit, staff tried not to make eye contact with the surveyors for fear of being asked a question. One nurse could barely state her name. Who were these creatures that instilled so much fear and terror? As a new nurse, I never experienced anything like this before. Maybe it was covered during orientation? Did we speak of it at nursing school? How about while studying for my board exam?

L. San Martin (✉)
University of Maryland Medical System, Baltimore, MD, USA
e-mail: Layla.SanMartin@umm.edu

R. Roberts-Turner, R. K. Shah (eds.), *Pocket Guide to Quality Improvement in Healthcare*,
https://doi.org/10.1007/978-3-030-70780-4_6

WHY DID I NOT PAY ATTENTION DURING ORIENTATION!!! What's my name again???

What did I do? Anything and everything I could not to get "apprehended." I took my break, pretended to take a very important care plan to the attending doctor, closed the curtain around my patient, and prayed they would come, go, and not interview me!

I was thankfully saved from this group of mythical all-knowing beings…this time. I slipped their attention, but they would be back, once every 3 years and others just like them with different titles, possibly on an annual occasion. Why? What for? Can't they see how busy we are? We do not have time for this!

As a new healthcare worker, a new nurse, I could not see the rationale for these surveys; every finding of "noncompliance" seemed insignificant, so what if the corridor was partially blocked with supplies? If you turned sideways you could squeeze past. Supplies everywhere? Yeah, we need them, why can't they be in cardboard boxes? Did it really matter that the refrigerator was off its "regular" temperature of 1 degree? Everyone knows frontline staff doesn't get enough breaks, so why can't I keep my drink at my workstation? Asking our supervisors "why" did not provide satisfaction; "BECAUSE I SAID SO" did not give us the momentum to follow these rules. Maybe they too didn't really understand the rationale for the rules?

So, why should we care? Healthcare regulation exists to ensure that any heath care facility or service offers a basic standard of care to protect patients and the staff who work there. It's not just about the structure of the building you work in, but it's also about staff education, staff qualifications, the culture of the organization, caring behaviors toward each other, and ensuring we are delivering the best care possible to our patients and families. No one ever wants to hurt anyone, and no one ever wants to get hurt in a healthcare facility while seeking care.

So, what is this chapter about? This chapter hopes to provide some answers to this regulatory mystery and demonstrate a "bigger picture" to healthcare regulatory compliance and why your role within this compliance is much bigger than you think. When I think back to my early years as a nurse, I wish I had this knowledge and appreciation of the regulatory aspect of healthcare delivery. A basic understanding is very important. Regulations not only keep your patients safe, they protect the organization, and if nothing else matters, YOUR professional license!

In this chapter we will review what healthcare regulation is, why you need to know it, why we need to have it, who the regulatory bodies are that you will deal with on a regular basis, what and how standards of care get written and submitted in the rule books, what role you can play to help your department prepare for a survey, how to talk to these mythical creatures (no special language certification needed), and how to support a state of continued survey readiness so that you are not scrambling 6 months, 2 weeks, and 1 day before they arrive.

What Is Healthcare Regulation and Accreditation and Why Should You Care?

Let's start at the top. There are many large health insurance companies that reimburse healthcare organizations for care delivered to their participating customers (patients). Medicare and Medicaid are federal and state programs that provide assistance to people that cannot afford their own health insurance due to low income and limited resources [4]. Regulation plays a major role in the healthcare industry and healthcare insurance coverage. These various regulatory bodies protect the public from numerous health risks and offer several programs for public health and welfare.

The US Department of Health and Human Services (HHS) is the part of the federal government responsible for administering the programs that deal with health and welfare. Healthcare regulation is primarily concerned with "enabling patient access to high quality, safe and effective care, and avoiding access to medical products and practices that are unsafe. When appropriately implemented, regulation ensures public health benefits and the safety of patients, healthcare workers, and the community" [7].

There are three main bodies of regulation within healthcare – the government, state, and accreditation bodies.

CMS and State Licensing: The Centers for Medicaid/Medicare Services

The Centers for Medicare and Medicaid (CMS) developed Conditions of Participation (CoPs) and Conditions for Coverage (CfCs) that healthcare organizations are required to meet to become certified and continue participating in the Medicare and Medicaid programs to receive reimbursement for care delivered. These health and safety standards are the foundation for improving quality and protecting the health and safety of the beneficiaries. These standards were created to evaluate and enforce safe healthcare practices across the United States [1]. In addition to meeting these requirements, the ability to achieve a high-quality, highly reliable organization demonstrates a heightened commitment to patient safety and excellence in delivery of care. None of this can be achieved without regulatory compliance and therefore becomes an essential element allowing healthcare facilities to be recognized as a lead competitor among other healthcare facilities and a top choice for patients seeking care.

This approval by the government can take form as certification and state licensing, which focuses on maintaining minimum standards to safeguard public health. The approval may be enough for some agencies; however, additional information may be required for reimbursement under other federal programs and health plans. Both state and federal regulations include quality management requirements, for example, licensing regulations in all states to require hospitals to have a system for measuring, evaluating, and reducing patient infection rates [1].

Healthcare facilities also have the option to voluntarily seek accreditation from other regulatory/accrediting bodies. CMS ensures that the standards of accreditation set forth by these bodies are equivalent to or exceed the Medicare standards through a process called "deeming." This voluntary process not only demonstrates a commitment to safe, high-quality care but also ensures that the organization is meeting or exceeding the CoPs, therefore, providing reimbursement for care delivered to Medicare and Medicaid beneficiaries. Many healthcare organizations are often both certified by government agencies and accredited by nongovernmental agencies for this purpose. CMS has granted several of these nongovernmental agencies' deemed status. Most evaluation processes involve surveys, reviewing client outcomes, as well as assessment of the structure of the organization and policies and processes used to provide care.

Other Regulatory Agencies

There are several other regulatory agencies with additional standards that a healthcare facility must also adhere to. These organizations include but are not limited to the Food and Drug Administration (FDA), Drug Enforcement Administration (DEA), National Committee for Quality Assurance (NCQA), Quality Improvement Organization (QIO), National Fire Protection Agency (NFPA), Occupational Safety & Health Administration (OSHA), and Department of Environmental Protection (DEP), among many others. All have different rules and standards to ensure the safety of the patient, families, staff, and the community. These agencies are major influences on the operation of healthcare organizations. Preparing for a visit from any one of these agencies requires the organization to self-assess their current compliance status and adapt appropriately.

Accreditation

Accreditation is a process of review that allows healthcare organizations to demonstrate their ability to meet regulatory requirements and standards established by a recognized accreditation organization and satisfy CMS requirements.

The Joint Commission (TJC)

The Joint Commission is a nonprofit, voluntary accreditation group that was established in 1951. This group accredits and certifies over 22,000 healthcare organizations and programs within the

United States. The Joint Commission accreditation and certifications are recognized nationwide as a symbol of quality, their standards are comprehensive and reflects an organization's commitment to meeting and exceeding certain performance standards [3].

Their surveys are conducted approximately every 3 years and investigate all aspects of the healthcare organization, including the physical plant, the entire delivery of care process, and the evaluation and quality improvement plan. An accreditation survey can last anywhere between 4 and 5 days, after which a report is generated with any findings. The organization then has a certain amount of time to challenge those findings if they believe they are practicing in compliance, and the final report is scored to indicate the severity of harm and how extensive the occurrence of the noncompliance is within the organization.

Any observations determined to place the public or patient in immediate jeopardy (serious threat to health and safety) can result in a preliminary denial of accreditation and termination of their Medicare/Medicaid certification if not resolved. Examples of immediate jeopardy can include the following:

- Facility's fire alarm system not working
- Fire doors not closing or latching appropriately
- No pre-procedural checklist completion verifying the right patient, correct procedure site, or side
- Ligature risks not addressed in areas caring for behavioral health patients

Unless the organization takes immediate action to rectify the situation, it may face removal of accreditation, removal of CMS certification, and potential closure. Once all observations have been reported and clarified, the organization has a designated amount of time to create and implement action plans to rectify the findings of noncompliance. Depending on the severity of the findings, the organization will need leadership involvement and an audit plan to monitor improvement. TJC may then return to monitor improvements and validate actions taken to resolve the noncompliance.

TJC also offers consultative services in between surveys, allowing the hospital access to consultants, "mock surveys," Standard Interpretation Group (where any regulatory questions can be submitted for professional response), and many tools to monitor compliance. This can be instrumental when working to achieve a state of continuous survey readiness.

Det Norske Veritas (DNV)

DNV (Det Norske Veritas) became the first alternative to the Joint Commission in 2008 for accreditation for hospitals. This non-profit organization has been in existence since 1864. Originating from Norway, this risk management company began operating in the United States in 1898, working with manufacturing and other industries on developing effective quality improvement processes to manage risk. The expansion into healthcare began in 2008 when they received their "deeming" authority. Currently, they provide accreditation for over 500 hospitals in the United States and are steadily becoming a strong alternative regulatory body to TJC. Their approach to healthcare regulation follows their standard model of operation extrapolated from other industries. DNV Surveys are conducted annually. Those institutions that meet the Medicare/Medicaid COP are accredited but are then guided toward improvement to meet the international standards, which reflect continuous quality improvement and customer satisfaction. Unlike the Joint Commission, DNV does not provide consultative services, nor does it provide prescriptive procedures or institutions. They state that their focus is to help organizations develop their own best practices by focusing on outcomes [2].

Competition among healthcare organizations is growing at an incredible rate. As the demand for high-quality services increases between healthcare organizations, the organizations that achieve recognition in the form of accreditation and certification will attract more consumers (including health insurance companies and their patients). If a patient gets injured or acquires a medical condition that they didn't have before they went to the hospital (e.g., the organization made an error or didn't prevent a situation from occurring; a patient developed a pressure injury, surgical site infection, or other hospital-acquired conditions), the hospital is responsible for covering the cost and can potentially face liability that can be made public and thus lose trust in their payers and local community.

What Is a Survey?

Regardless of what regulatory/accreditation organization comes to the healthcare facility you work in, the survey process will follow a similar process and agenda. Surveyors typically turn up at the front desk and announce their arrival, whether expected or unexpected. The regulatory department of the facility will greet them, verify their identity, and coordinate all survey efforts from a central location. A notification is sent to all areas under the organizational hospital license being surveyed. Typically, the surveyors open with the reason for their visit, whether it is for the facility's recertification, reaccreditation, a response to a complaint, or to tour a newly renovated or constructed area. Regardless of their agenda, all areas and employees of the hospital must be notified and prepare their areas accordingly in the event the surveyor wants to tour the area and interview staff.

Surveys can be anywhere from several hours to a week-long event. Depending on the survey type, the surveyors may review all elements of care related to the purpose of their visit:

- The physical structure of the buildings.
- Safety of the environment where care is delivered.
- Types of care administered to various patient populations served.
- Types of documentation recorded related to the care delivered.
- Competency and credentials of the employees working within the facility.
- Organizational leadership structure.
- The temperature the dishes are washed.

- The cleanliness of the pots and pans the food is cooked in.
- Even the PH level of the rice we serve in the cafeteria. Every element is assessed.

Regardless of their purpose that day, even if it is to look at a newly renovated area within one wing of the building, they still need to get there. If while the surveyor is being escorted to that location, they see something out of compliance, then they must investigate and write a report citing for the noncompliance. Each citation or finding is added to a final report and results in the facility writing action plans to resolve the issue, which may entail amending an old or writing a new policy, educating staff, and evaluating compliance via auditing. Each finding may result in a fine; a resurvey; if particularly severe and puts the safety of the patient or staff in jeopardy, loss of accreditation or certification; or worse case, closure of the facility.

How do we make sure that doesn't happen? Each agency or accreditation organization has published standards of care or conditions that each hospital must meet. These are the rules and regulations that every healthcare facility must adhere to in order to remain open, functioning, and receive payment. Each regulation or standard is written to enhance the quality of care, keep the patient safe, and to prevent harm. Every hospital or healthcare organization typically has a patient safety officer and regulatory department who are fluent in interpreting these standards and help facilitate compliance with each one. These standards are reviewed and updated a couple of times a year, and each healthcare organization must understand and ensure the elements are met.

Survey Preparation

In order to be ready for these surveys, preparation is key. If you find yourself scrambling weeks before a survey is due, your efforts may be inadequate and lead to many non-compliant observations. A constant state of readiness must be achieved in order to be prepared for a survey at any time. As previously described, many surveys are unannounced, so healthcare organizations don't typically know precisely when they will occur. We may have anywhere from an 18-month to a 60-day window. Preparing a facility for such an event can take a significant amount of time. Each department, unit, clinic, specialty area must understand the requirements and ensure that the delivery of care, evidence of that care delivered, and their care environment support compliance. Each survey has a specific set of documents required for the surveyors to review this can include but is not limited to the following:

- Organizational charts
- List of offsite facilities under the organizational license
- Policies and procedures
- Standard work or practice guidelines
- Medical staff bylaws (rules for providers to practice) competency and education review
- Infection control plans
- Various committee meeting minutes (patient safety, medical executive committee, quality committee)
- Quality measurements on specific aspects of care such as surgical site infection rates, restraint and seclusion practices, and contracts with outside vendors (agency staff, services)
- Restrain and seclusion logs
- Staffing sheets
- Patient isolation lists
- Operating room schedules
- Hospital grievance/complaint log
- Employee files and credentialing: If you are a healthcare employee, your human resource file may get reviewed. Surveyors will be looking for validation of the following:
  - License
  - Certifications
  - Orientation to the facility
  - Specific job requirements of your role
  - Continuing education

If you are a frontline staff member, your patient may get selected for a chart review, and although they are looking at every aspect of care, they may want to ask you questions about your patient. They want you to "know the patient's story" and demonstrate you are delivering required care and documenting it appropriately.

It is good practice to ensure you are delivering care according to the policies and procedures of the facility and the state licensing board you are registered with. Keeping abreast of revised standards of care is important not just to protect your patient and the organization but also to your professional license. Keep up to date with best practices, and make sure you are meeting all your certification and relicensure requirements. Surveyors and certification agencies will spot check your continuing education completion, so keep copies!

Survey Etiquette

Many people often clam up when being approached by a surveyor. From the beginning of this chapter, you can see that I too tried to do everything but sit in front of a surveyor. As mentioned, some people cannot even state their name let alone respond to a question regarding the care of a patient. The biggest trick is to just take a deep breath. They just want to know that you are competent for your role and are delivering care according to the facility's guidelines. Surveyors can and will want to talk to anyone in the facility, nurses, doctors, technicians, environmental staff, dietary staff, therapists, leaders, and even the patient and families themselves. They want to know the story of the care you are delivering, that you understand your role and responsibility in the process, and for you to "brag" about yourself. Show them that you care.

It is understood that you may not know all the answers to their questions and that's okay! What they are looking for is that you know who and where your resources are. It is very rare that a surveyor would be unaccompanied by an organizational staff member. Almost always, they will have an escort and a scribe (staff member who takes notes) accompany them. It is their job to direct the surveyor to the correct unit and take notes on elements discussed. The unit supervisor or person in charge will meet them on the unit and be able to answer most questions regarding the running of the unit and the processes of care delivered. There will be certain questions that are repeatedly asked throughout the survey that ALL staff members are expected to know:

- How to use a fire extinguisher using the PASS acronym: Pull, Aim, Squeeze, Sweep.
- Process when you discover a fire [6] or when to evacuate an area using the RACE acronym: Rescue, Alarm, Contain, Extinguish or Evacuate [5].
- Emergency evacuation routes for the unit.
- Who is permitted to operate the medical gas shutoff valves within the unit during an emergency?
- How to call for help?
- Where to find material safety data sheets when there has been a chemical spill?

These is critical knowledge that you need to know. All these elements are typically reviewed during orientation to the facility, and each regulatory "mock" survey or practice session that your regulatory department conducts can go over this information along with other common issues/findings.

Continued Survey Readiness: *Surveys, Audits, and Tracers—OH MY!!*

Let's talk about ways to keep you updated and ready for a regulatory survey.

Use practice runs (mock tracers) and stay informed by your organization's regulatory team to boost your compliance knowledge. These are the times that should be used for educational purposes. It is not a punitive practice, better to not know during a "mock survey" than on the day of the actual survey. Your regulatory team can educate you on the rationale of various standards and practices. "BECAUSE I SAID SO" (as much as people love saying it) is no longer acceptable, so ask lots of questions, and find out who or where your resources are.

So, what are some of the most common findings during a survey? Over the many years I have been practicing in healthcare and having taken part in many different types of surveys, trends of noncompliance do tend to reappear over and over. The majority are what we like to call "low-hanging fruit," simple observations that are easy to fix but seem to repeatedly raise their ugly heads, whether during a practice survey by the organizations, regulatory staff or during a real-time survey. These little issues accumulate into a big deal and seem to reappear month after month and year after year. Some time ago, surveyors would only cite an organization if it found repetitive issues across the organization during the survey such as stained ceiling tiles in three separate areas, failure to document pain reassessment within the permitted time frame in three patient charts, or emergency call bells not freely hanging in more than three patient bathrooms. The "trend of three" are the ones that used to get you a citation. Today, a surveyor will find an organization out of compliance with just one of those occurrences. Below are more examples of common non-compliant findings:

- Expired supplies
  - Expired supplies are a common problem. Would you want an expired supply used on you? Although a few days out of date seems insignificant, the expiration date is there for a reason. The supply has been tested and an amount of time designated for that supply to function at its most effective. Most of us have experienced spoiled milk or food in the refrigerator. It tastes bad and will most likely give you a stomachache, so you know not to drink or eat it if the expiration date has passed. When medical supplies expire, there can be serious consequences to the patient. When blood test tubes are expired, the additives in that tube could spoil and become less efficient, which can cause an unreliable test result. Additives in an intravenous bag of fluid can lose its potency. CPR electro pads lose their conductivity and don't

show an accurate heart rhythm or distribute electricity appropriately to correct abnormal heart rhythm. Expired supplies occur due to a number of reasons: (1) the unit/department orders too many and doesn't have the regular use for it, so it sits on a shelf for too long; (2) staff who restock the supply rooms do not rotate the supplies from the back to the front, so supplies in the back never get used first and therefore expire; (3) multi-packs are opened and not dated or timed, interfering with the integrity of the product which then becomes time-sensitive (e.g., multi-pack IV fluids, glucose monitoring strips, quality control solutions).

Many staff like to create their own specialty packs for tasks, IV start kits, trauma kits, wound care supplies, and then stow them away in secret drawers of a unit. Surveyors will find them. Akin to security canines at an airport, they will find them, and 9 times out of 10, an element of the kit will be expired. The solution? Weekly/monthly checks to make sure that supply amounts match the need, that staff are rotating supplies when restocking, and that staff using supply carts and kits check them regularly and use or replace items before they expire. Every surveyor will typically check one supply from the front, middle, and back of the storage container to ensure supplies are compliant.

- Blocked egress (corridors or doors blocked with clutter)

  Storage space is always a challenge in every healthcare facility. There is just not enough room for beds, chairs, lifts, carts, etc. Often equipment is left in the corridor of the unit, and until you need a clear corridor when running for your life in an emergency, you don't realize it's a problem. Anything stationary and not in use for over 30 minutes is generally considered blocked egress and demonstrates noncompliance with life safety measurements. Items that are always considered in use would be an isolation cart outside a patient's room who is currently in isolation (patients must have an order for this, the surveyor WILL check) or a code cart that must be within an acceptable distance from the patient care area. Computers on wheels are permitted if you are currently using it; otherwise, if after 30 minutes it remains unused, the surveyor will consider its storage non-compliant. Some newer hospitals have larger/wider corridors that permit storage on equipment to one side of the corridor, however for the majority of older hospitals which were built according to older guidelines, the corridors are too small and must remain clear.

- Blocked emergency equipment
  - So, where to put all this equipment from the corridor? Unfortunately, it is often stored in front of emergency equipment such as a fire extinguisher, fire alarm, or fire pull. It can be understood that healthcare staff see these emergency elements constantly and it becomes part of the "decoration," but again like a blocked egress, when you need to use the emergency equipment, time is of the essence, and trying to move a cart or a stack of chairs blocking access to this life-saving equipment can spell injury to the staff member who is trying to access it and possible harm to the staff or patient member who require it. Maintaining a clear path to this equipment is necessary and should always be monitored. A procedural area such as the operating room is a repeat offender for this. They have so many large pieces of equipment that must be on standby in the event that they need it, and that often will sit outside the operating room for several hours unintentionally blocking egress, the emergency alarm pulls, shutoff handles, and fire extinguishers.
  - Patient bathroom call bells can also be problematic. Often these emergency alarms can be found wrapped around the handrail in the patient bathroom. If the patient falls and pulls on the alarm cord, it will not alarm because the cord is then trapped and will not activate (it is wrapped around the handrail). Who is the perpetrator? Well it can be anyone. Patients and their visitors may play with it while using the restroom, and environmental service staff can wrap it around the handrail as not to get it wet when they are mopping the floors. It is not done on purpose but can have a

significant impact on the safety of your patient, so make it a good practice habit, and periodically check your patient bathrooms to make sure it is free from any obstacle.

- Outside shipping boxes
  - Shipping boxes! All supplies come in them. The majority of supplies are de-boxed in the facility's loading dock; however, large items/multiple items may find their way to your patient care area and either be stored on the floor or on carts in their original cardboard boxes. What's so bad about that? Well, cardboard is a fuel source, so if any fire broke out, it has something additional to burn. These supplies have traveled from a warehouse, on a ship, truck, and now your unit. Nobody really knows the cleanliness of the storage area it was prepared or transport it was shipped on. Cardboard is a very hospitable place for critters to stow away. No one wants a rodent living on their unit or several bugs running around. The infection control and disease transmission risk are a huge concern, but this is something we can attempt to limit. Patients bring in their own belongings and therefore can bring in their own fair share of unwanted pets too! Pest control services is a routine contract service for every healthcare organization. However, if we want to reduce the risk, then measures must be put into place. This is why it is important that all outside shipping boxes (if they make it to your unit) are emptied and removed.

Two urban legends come to mind when I write this. One is where a pallet of supplies was delivered to a large patient care area during the night shift. As the supplies were delivered on a small internal forklift, the pallet was set down in the corridor, and staff began to unload and restock the clean supply room. As they got to the bottom of the pallet, they inadvertently disturbed a bat who had tucked himself away in a corner of the pallet, and he began to fly around the unit until a staff member managed to capture the poor creature. The second event was in a postoperative recovery room where a mother was watching her child recover from surgery only to report to the nurse that there was a very tiny bird flying around their room. To the nurse's horror, it was in fact a rather large flying insect. Containing her horror, the nurse proceeded to catch the bug in a trash bag and dispose appropriately. Some situations cannot be prevented but can be minimized.

- Room/refrigerator/freezer temperature checks
  - This is another common finding. Daily temperature checks are required whenever storing food, medication, sterile supplies, specimens, warming blankets, or liquids in certain care areas. Temperature ranges vary according to what you are storing in that room or appliance, and any deviation out of the approved ranges can have significant implications to the integrity of the product or equipment. If the temperatures are manually checked, the log sheet must be completed daily. It is understood that shifts can get busy, but there must be a backup plan to ensure these temperature checks are monitored. Many organizations have moved to remote monitoring if the central monitoring hub detects a fluctuation or consistent temperature change out of the approved range, a report is generated and sent to the unit, and action must be taken. Unfortunately, this communication can be misinterpreted. Remotely monitoring a temperature does not mean that another department is aware; it can simply mean that a computer detected and generated the report and that it is the end user's responsibility to act. If your unit or area has stored sterile supplies, medication/food refrigerators, freezers, or warmers, then make sure you understand who monitors the temperatures and what actions must be taken to correct it. This can be particularly problematic for an organization's offsite outpatient facility that does not open for business on a weekend. Many refrigerators contain vaccines and medications that still require remote monitoring. Notification of an out-of-range temperature is often sent to pharmacy to come and remove the supplies so as not to ruin their integrity. Some medication

refrigerator spaces and storage rooms can be small, and the machine that delivers the medication generates a significant amount of heat. If there is not enough air space and air circulation, the room can easily heat up putting undue burden on the refrigerator causing it to fail or the room to exceed permitted temperature ranges for supply integrity. Digital thermometers often have their own calibration needs, and a small expiration date can be found on the back of them. Make sure these dates are checked, or the integrity of the thermometer themselves can come into question and thus question the validity of the temperature recording.

One other observation to point out is regarding cleanliness of the refrigerator and freezers themselves. Regardless of what these devices are keeping cool or frozen, cleanliness and function is important. Over-frosted freezers can again compromise its ability to function or even close the door. Unit leaders should identify who is responsible for cleaning and checking them on a routine basis.

- Stained/broken ceiling tiles
  - Every building at some point will have a plumbing leak. Stained ceiling tiles indicate a leak of some sort and will require attention. If your facility is following its policy and procedures appropriate to resolve the issue, the surveyor will acknowledge compliance. This typically means that a work order has been placed to fix the leak and replace the tile. If you can produce this document, then the surveyor typically goes about their business. However, if the work order had been submitted beyond the stated response time in the engineering department's policy, then this becomes an observation of noncompliance. The same for any broken tiles or ones that have holes in them. This affects its fire integrity (ability to delay the spread of the fire) and can become a fire risk.
- Wall penetrations
  - Like the broken ceiling tiles, any deep scrapes chipped paint or holes in the wall also need to be submitted for repair to the

facility's department. This again can become a fire risk as well as an infection control issue. Wall penetrations not only alter the integrity of a firewall but also are a great place for little creatures to escape, breed, and plot their infestation.

- Preventative maintenance
  - All equipment utilized in the delivery of patient care must be logged, accounted for, and maintained. There are thousands of different types of equipment that must be checked and inspected on a routine basis to ensure its function and safety for use. All equipment needs to be logged in order, so if a recall was announced by the biomedical team, the organization can quickly retrieve, remove, and/or replace it. In the event of an emergency, a quick inventory check can ascertain how many pieces of equipment (such as ventilators) an organization has and how many more may need to be acquired to meet the demand. Each piece of machinery requires maintenance checks and will be placed on a schedule for service. Once the equipment has passed inspection, a sticker will be placed on the item that states either the day it was inspected or when the next date of inspection is due. It is good practice to check these stickers when using the equipment as one or two may have slipped past the due date due to them being inpatient use at the time of inspection. If that is the case, the item should be removed, tagged appropriately, and stored in a location for pickup.
- Holiday decorations

  This is always a challenge. No patient wants to be in hospital during the holidays or during any celebration. Staff are always trying to lift their patient's spirits by decorating units. This can be problematic as too much paper decoration, electrical lights, and decorations hanging from the ceiling pose a fire and safety threat. Hospitals are a highly combustible environment, enriched with oxygen pumping through the walls and storing all types of flammable chemicals; the organization always needs to minimize the risk of fire. Fires have occurred, holiday trees have caught on fire due to too many electrical lights, patients have tripped from decorations being wrapped around corridor handrails, and IV fluids have been pulled out of patient arms from getting caught in ceiling decorations. Not to say organizations can't decorate, it just needs to be controlled and approved by the organization's life safety committee.

- Documentation

The majority of what has been discussed references the environment of patient care. Another area that is always reviewed, and is often missing elements, is documentation of care. All care delivered should be noted in the patient's record. The patient's medical record is the evidence that care is provided, and if you are ever ordered to attend a court case or a deposition where patient care is questioned (sometimes 5–7 years after the care was provided), all you will have to rely on is the documentation you completed, as chances are you may not remember every patient encounter you are involved in. Commonly missing pieces of documentation are as follows:

- Consent for hospital treatment
  - All patients should sign a consent to treatment when seeking care in a facility
  - All surgical patients should have a complete informed procedural consent form
- History and physical updates
  - The provider completes this and specific updates that are required for certain care practices
- Plans of care
  - Every patient needs a plan of care that is based on the problems identified upon admission. This plan must be reviewed daily. Patient goals are established, and progress is assessed on their ability to meet these goals. Unfortunately, not every plan of care identifies all the patient goals. Often, pain, learning barriers, and wound care plans can be missing. The plan of care should be an interdisciplinary team approach; both provider and bedside staff are responsible for reviewing and updating the plan. Sometimes these responsibilities can be misunderstood and the plan left incomplete.

- Assessment/reassessment times in the patient record
  - Assessment and reassessments are treatment based. Skin assessment can be required per shift – neurological assessments every 4 hours or per physician order. Pain assessment/reassessment depends on whether the intervention is pharmacological (medically treated) or non-pharmacological (heat, aromatherapy, healing touch, ice, distraction, meditation application). Assessment and reassessment should be based on your organizations policy and procedure or standard work practices. Often the surveyor will compare the care delivered to what the organization states is care delivered within their own guidelines. Most policy and procedures are based on evidence-based care and best practices. The organization has done their homework and developed their practices on what works and what works best, comparing to other similar organization's practices and their outcomes (these are the quality improvement measures that I mentioned earlier). This is an area that you may see as opportunity for improvement and in the future become interested in improving.
- Medication orders and administration
  - Administering medications can be one of the most dangerous tasks a healthcare worker has to practice. There is a long history of medication errors that have ended in a patient's death or permanent harm. Medication orders must be written according to specific guidelines, cross checked, and approved by several staff and pharmacists including the person administering them. If you are not familiar with a medication that you need to administer, do your due diligence and look it up. Ask yourself, what are the side effects? Does it interact with another medication your patient is taking? Is your patient allergic to it? Above all, follow the organizations process to safe medication administration.
  - Technology is making it easier to administer the correct medication to the correct patient. Technology, however, is only as good as its user. Healthcare workers are well known to create "work-arounds" or "shortcuts" to practice more

> efficiently, but this could possibly lead to huge error and thus lead to severe patient harm. Remember that these processes are in place for a reason…to keep everyone safe! One example I can share is when I worked in a very busy patient care unit on a night shift. I had two patients with the same last name in the same room (I know, what are the chances? It would probably never happen today). Both went for a procedure during the day, and when they came back their beds had been switched but remained in the same room. Coming from four nights off, I was not familiar with the patients and in the middle of several admission and discharges went about administering medications. The medication administration record (MAR) at the time was on paper and located on the medication cart. I dispensed their medications into a cup, took the paper MAR with me, and checked their names, focusing on their last names. I was about to hang an IV antibiotic treatment when I noticed the patient looking at the IV. I stopped, checked his arm band again against the MAR, and realized to my horror that the MAR did not correspond to the patient's medical record number. I was about to give him his roommate's medication! The patients had been switched, but their records were never switched in the MAR binder. I will never forget that ice-cold wave of nausea I felt knowing that I could have given him the wrong medication. From that day forward, I triple-checked every medication I ever administered no matter how busy I was.

All these rules and regulations were created for a reason. Either patient harm occurred or it almost did, and every healthcare organization wants to try to prevent harm at all costs. Every employee is counted on to do their part, ask questions when unsure, practice in a safe manner according to the organization's policy and procedure, and above all speak up when something does not seem right.

Let's Wrap This Up!

Basically, there are three main groups of regulatory bodies that have rules and regulations that hospitals must adhere to in order to safely care for patients and receive payment. These regulatory bodies will pay a visit to each healthcare organization either because certification or accreditation is desired, they received a complaint, or there was an upgrade or addition to the environment. Regardless of the reason, any noncompliance found against these regulations results in a fine and possible closure if not resolved. These surveys are a BIG DEAL. They occur to ensure the safety of the public and the staff who work there. Achievement and sustainment of accreditation and certification demonstrate a commitment to high-quality care and safe patient and play a major supportive role in the quality improvement process. Everyone has a part to play. It's okay not to know all the answers to the questions they may ask you, but you do need to know where you can find those answers, so pay attention during orientation, ask lots of questions to your organization's regulatory department, and keep up to date with your role and responsibilities including continuing education. Do not take "BECAUSE I SAID SO" for an answer!

References

1. CMS.gov. 2020. Conditions for coverage & conditions of participation. https://www.cms.gov/Regulations-and-Guidance/Legislation/CFCsAndCoPs. Accessed 30 June 2020.
2. DNV. 2020. Hospital accreditation. https://www.dnvglhealthcare.com/accreditations/hospital-accreditation. Accessed 30 June 2020.
3. The Joint Commission. 2020. History of the joint commission. https://www.jointcommission.org/about-us/facts-about-the-joint-commission/history-of-the-joint-commission/. Accessed 30 June 2020.
4. Medicare.gov. n.d. How is Medicare funded. https://www.medicare.gov/about-us/how-is-medicare-funded. Accessed 30 June 2020.
5. ECRI Institute. 2020. Responding to Fires in Areas of Oxygen use. http://www.mdsr.ecri.org/summary/detail.aspx?doc_id=8164. Accessed 30 June 2020.
6. Occupational Safety and Health Administration. 2020. Evacuation plans and procedures eTool. https://www.osha.gov/SLTC/etools/evacuation/portable_use.html. Accessed 30 June 2020.
7. World Health Organization. 2020. Regulations. https://www.who.int/medical_devices/safety/en/. Accessed 30 June 2020.

7 Infection Prevention and Control: Applying Common Sense to Everyday Practice

Xiaoyan Song and Jeffrey Li

Background

The concept of infection control stemmed from observations that Dr. Ignaz Semmelweis made about 200 years ago in 1847 [1]. As the house staff officer in one of two obstetric clinics at the University of Vienna Allgemeines Krankenhaus (General Hospital), Semmelweis observed that patients in one clinic suffered much higher maternal mortality rates than the other, mostly attributed to puerperal fever. He noticed that doctors and medical students often went directly to the delivery suite after performing autopsies and had an odor on their hands despite handwashing with soap and water before entering the clinic. As a result, Semmelweis recommended that hands be scrubbed in a chlorinated lime solution before every patient contact and after leaving autopsies. Following the implementation of this measure, the mortality rate fell by 80% and remained low. Semmelweis is

X. Song
Office of Infection Control/Epidemiology, Children's National Hospital, Washington, DC, USA
e-mail: xsong@cnmc.org

J. Li (✉)
Independent Researcher, Clarksville, MD, USA

R. Roberts-Turner, R. K. Shah (eds.), *Pocket Guide to Quality Improvement in Healthcare*,
https://doi.org/10.1007/978-3-030-70780-4_7

viewed as the founding father of hand hygiene; his intervention is also a model of how to use epidemiologically-driven strategies to prevent infection [1–3].

In the hundred years following Semmelweis' breakthrough, medicine and public health have significantly advanced to meet the needs of human beings. With the development of bacteriology, European discoveries such as Pasteur's rabies treatment, diphtheria antitoxin, and typhoid vaccination were quickly introduced into the United States. By World War II, emerging new drugs, especially penicillin, took modern medicine to a new level. The introduction of the polio vaccine in the 1950s, following a massive research effort, was a thrilling public and scientific event. Recent decades have also witnessed substantial progress in immunization and vaccination against influenza, measles, allergies, and other diseases.

These remarkable excitements have been mixed with sobering experiences. The epidemic of penicillin-resistant *Staphylococcus aureus* infections that occurred during the 1950s ravaged hospital nurseries. It captured the public's attention and highlighted the importance of implementing techniques to prevent infections in healthcare settings [4]. In the mid-twentieth century, some surgeons, microbiologists, and infectious disease physicians began to focus their studies on the epidemiology and control of infections in hospital settings. By the 1960s, hospital-based infection control efforts had been established in scattered hospitals throughout the United States. The number of hospitals with infection control programs increased substantially during the 1970s, and infection control programs were present in almost every US hospital by the early 1990s.

To date, although healthcare facilities and infection control experts have made significant progress in preventing some types of infections, there is still significant work that needs to occur. Each year in the United States, at least 2.8 million people contract an antibiotic-resistant infection, and more than 35,000 people die. It's important that each healthcare worker understands proper infection control procedures, for patient health and their own health.

The role of infection control and public health cannot be understated. We are currently the midst of a once-in-a-lifetime crisis. The COVID-19 pandemic has turned the lives of millions of people upside down and will likely have implications on our society as a whole in the coming years. The healthcare industry is no exception; COVID-19's infectivity and severity have increasingly brought infectious control measures under scrutiny and rocketed infection control practices into the public's eye. As infection control specialists, it is our duty now more than ever to ensure everyone, both inside and outside hospitals, correctly follows infection control measures.

Purpose of Infection Control

The purpose of an infection control program in a hospital is to prevent or stop the spread of infections among patients.

People often think that because hospitals cure illnesses and make people feel better, they are safe places. It's quite the opposite: hospitals are very dangerous *because* they cure illnesses and make people feel better. When a person feels ill and walks into a hospital seeking medical care, they do not know what disease they have nor its infectivity. Unless hospitals put infection control and other safety measures in place, being in a hospital can place one at risk for infectious disease. Besides this, hospitals are busy places, and many people, processes, supplies, devices, and spaces are involved in a patient's care. When one of these components fails to comply with infection control measures, patients can be at risk of acquiring an infection that is unwanted, unnecessary, and often avoidable.

These infections, whether they are acquired in a hospital or developed as a result of seeking medical care, are known as healthcare-associated infections (HAIs). HAIs are a type of medical error and are harmful to patients, hospitals, and society at large. They are associated with both extra care and additional costs for care. Despite treatment, many lives are still lost to HAIs, jeopardizing hospitals' reputations and placing them at risk for lawsuits.

History did not record who first understood or recognized HAIs, but by the 1960s, hospital-based clinicians and Centers for Disease Control and Prevention (CDC) epidemiologists were beginning to tackle HAIs. Common public health strategies were applied to build an HAI prevention system that focused on systematic surveillance to identify HAIs. This system implemented ongoing analysis of surveillance data to recognize potential problems, application of epidemic investigation techniques to epidemics and endemic HAIs, and implementation of hospital-wide interventions to protect patients, staff, and visitors.

Everyday, approximately one in every thirty-one patients in the United States contracts at least one infection associated with his or her hospital care, underscoring the need for improvements in patient care practices in US healthcare facilities. While great progress has been made, more still needs to be done to prevent healthcare-associated infections in a variety of settings. Today, hospitals are expected to implement "zero-tolerance" policies toward HAIs into the culture and care of their patients and are incentivized to reduce HAIs and improve patient outcomes. Hospitals are required to support a well-organized infection control program to develop, institute, and advance infection control practices in a hospital routine process – the result being markedly improved care and outcomes for patients.

Scope of Infection Control Practice

Infection control practice is patient-first; it includes every individual visiting or working in a hospital and anything that interacts with a patient.

Such a broad scope of service is defined by the chain of infection, the basic principle behind infection transmission, and the foundation on which infection prevention is built (Fig. 7.1). The chain of infection has six components: an *infectious agent*, a *reservoir* that hosts the agent, a *portal of exit* from the reservoir to the environment, a *mode of transmission* through the environment, and a *portal of entry* into the *susceptible host*. For infection to spread, all six links must work together unbroken. As such,

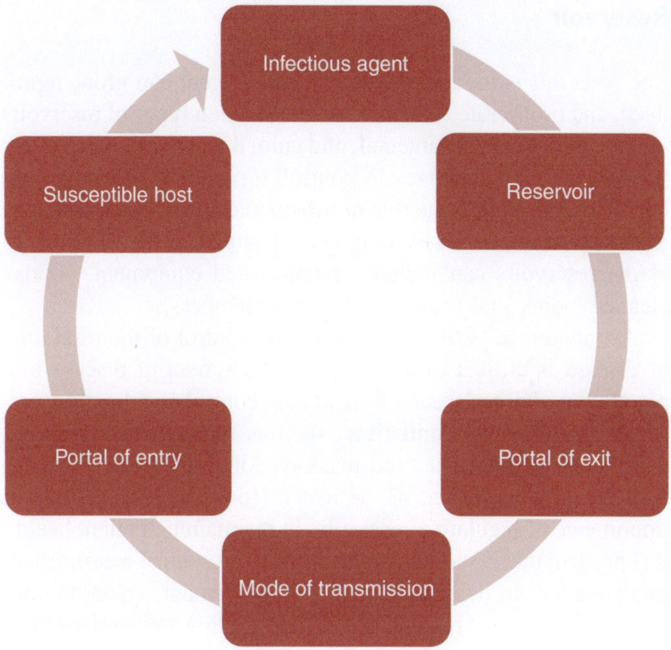

Fig. 7.1 The chain of infection

infection control is about the prevention of these components and the breaking of one or more links in the chain.

Infectious Agent

Infectious agents come in many different shapes and sizes. There are five major types of agents – bacteria, viruses, fungi, protozoa, and helminths. Bacteria, viruses, and fungi account for nearly all hospital-acquired infections and healthcare-setting outbreaks. When considering infectious disease, the infectious agent is often the first component of the chain of transmission that comes to mind. Generally, for an infection to occur, the agent must be present in the susceptible host; however, the efficacy of the agent in causing disease is influenced by other factors such as pathogenicity and infectivity [5].

Reservoir

The reservoir is the location in which an agent can grow, reproduce, and proliferate. The three most common types of reservoirs include human, environmental, and animal reservoirs. Each poses its own unique challenges in controlling and stopping the incidence of disease; it is the role of infection control specialists to be aware of the reservoirs existing in a hospital at any given time. In HAIs, reservoirs can include contaminated equipment, poorly-cleaned rooms, and visitors and family members.

As mentioned before, awareness and control of the reservoirs of disease is critical in undermining the spread of disease in a population and healthcare. Part of this control is reliant on personal accountability; initiatives, such as frequent handwashing, equipment maintenance, and mask-wearing, are entirely dependent on the compliance of the users. However, considering the importance of regulating reservoirs in maintaining patient health, it is prudent that reservoir-targeted infection control measures are implemented. In delivering quality improvement, infection control specialists must recognize clinical variation and work to capitalize on their hospital's strengths and work on their weaknesses.

Portal of Exit

The portal of exit is any method by which an agent exits its reservoir. In the case of human reservoirs, an infectious agent can exit through open wounds, aerosols, and splatter of body fluids including coughing, sneezing, and saliva.

Mode of Transmission

The mode of transmission is the method with which an agent leaves its reservoir until it reaches the next susceptible host. Mode of transmission can be broadly classified into direct and indirect transmission. Direct transmission includes direct contact and droplet spread, whereas indirect transmission includes airborne, vehicleborne, and vectorborne diseases.

Contact transmission occurs when there is direct skin-on-skin exposure. While droplet spread may sound similar to airborne transmission, droplets typically have a lower range and shorter infectious lifespan than airborne agents. Airborne agents can remain suspended in the air on droplet nuclei or dust or as an aerosol for much longer times. Vehicleborne illnesses are borne by inanimate media, such as surfaces, food, and bodily fluids. In contrast, vectors are animate carriers of disease; vectors may transmit disease solely through mechanical means or they may harbor growth and proliferation.

Portal of Entry

The portal of entry is how an agent enters a susceptible host. Modern healthcare employs many types of invasive devices and procedures to treat patients. When a central line, tube, or drain is inserted in a patient to either inject life-saving medication or to drain unwanted fluids out of the body, the procedure creates a potential portal of entry. Portals of entry are also created at surgery sites when the skin is deliberately opened. An infection can occur at any moment in a patient's care when an infectious agent enters through any one of these portals.

Susceptible Host

The final link in the chain of transmission is the host. The susceptibility of a host to infection is dependent on multiple factors, including genetics, environment, and physical health. Patients whose condition requires medical attention are often more predisposed to infection. HAIs pose a high risk to patients of all ages and demographics. As such, it is important that the previous five links in the chain are broken before it reaches the susceptible host.

Strategies to Break the Chain of Infectionz

A hierarchy of controls is shown in Fig. 7.2 based upon the effectiveness of various strategies that have been developed to break the chain of infection. These strategies include elimination, substitution, engineering controls, administrative controls, and personal protective equipment. Elimination refers to physically removing hazards, including infectious agents, harmful behaviors, and others. If a hazard is unable to be removed, replacing it with less harmful agents (substitution) and physically separating hazards from people (engineering control) are also options. Sometimes, simply changing the way that people work reduces hazard risk (administrative control). The least effective means of handling hazards is to use personal protective equipment (PPE), used when people must work in environments with uncontrollable hazards. Despite its low efficacy, PPE is also the most intuitive

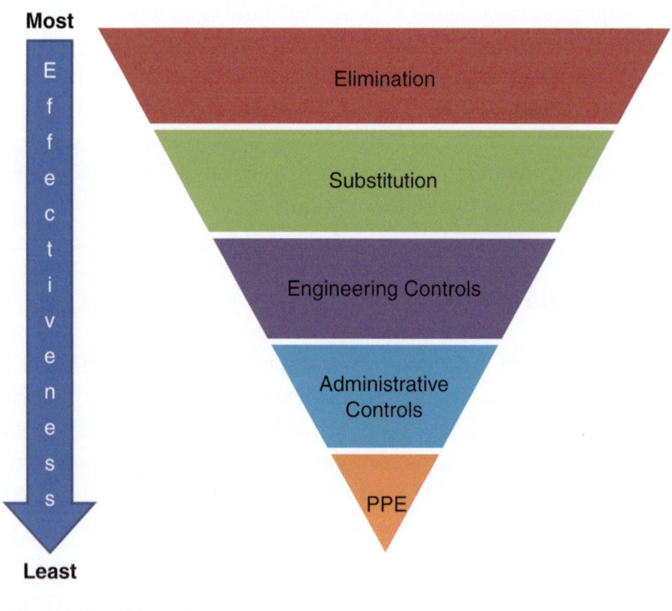

Fig. 7.2 The hierarchy of controls

way to make people feel safe: placing a physical barrier between a user and their environment.

Elimination

Hand hygiene may be the best example of using elimination strategies to prevent infections. As Semmelweis demonstrated hundreds of years ago, clean hands save lives. Hands are a natural reservoir of millions of microorganisms; some of these are commensal microbes that are beneficial to humans. For example, *Staphylococcus epidermidis*, the most common commensal skin flora, typically lives harmlessly on the skin. However, *Staphylococcus epidermidis* is also the number one cause of bloodstream infections in patients with a central venous catheter (CVC) [6]. CVC insertion creates a portal of entry that opens directly into a patient's bloodstream. When improperly sanitized hands handle catheters, microorganisms on the hands can inadvertently migrate into a patient's blood, causing life-threatening bloodstream infections.

Furthermore, when staff members touch medical devices or environments, their hands can be contaminated with environmental microbes. Hands that are not sufficiently cleaned between patients and between environments can become dangerous mediums, transmitting infectious agents from one patient to the other or from nonviable environments to humans. Besides the hands of healthcare providers, those of patients and visitors can become contaminated with microorganisms as well. When patients fail to wash their hands before eating or drinking, they can contract infections such as gastroenteritis or *Clostridium difficile*. Even when healthcare workers uphold the highest standards of infection control, the many other moving gears in the hospital machine may still fail.

Another example of when elimination works is the process of cleaning, disinfection, and sterilization. Microbes are ubiquitous elements of environments and human life. However, when microbes enter bodily sites that are meant to be sterile, like the blood or the heart, infections may occur. Hence, during many surgical and nonsurgical procedures, instruments that contact patients are expected to be microbe-free, to minimize infection risk. The elimination of microbial elements from these instruments is achieved through sterilization, a process that has been embraced in modern medicine. However, surgery predated sterilization by a full 600 years. The principles of asepsis and anesthesia were introduced in the mid-1800s by Joseph Lister, who invented the basic tenets of antisepsis and prevention of wound infection by eliminating germs on instruments, dressings, hands, and everything else in contact with wounds [7]. These principles of asepsis remain in use to this day. Failure to eliminate microbes from instruments almost certainly causes infection, as evidenced by many outbreaks reported in hospitals [8]. An analysis of nosocomial outbreaks between 1980 and 1990 found contaminated medical products and devices to be the number one cause of infection outbreaks! The analysis also demonstrated an ominous trend: in just 5 years, outbreaks caused by these devices and products increased by 50%. Decades later, hospitals continue to struggle with meeting safety standards on reprocessing used instruments and improving from HAI clusters and outbreaks [9–11].

Aside from large equipment, standard medical supplies, such as saline water, antiseptic agent, heparin flush, and more, have all been implicated in infection outbreaks [12–15]. Every incident sounds the alarm, reminding people of the importance of sterility throughout the entire patient care delivery process. This delivery process begins outside of the healthcare facility when a product is manufactured in a factory, continues when a product is stored and handled inside a healthcare facility, and ends when a product reaches a patient. Every person, every product, and every step in this process count toward safe care.

Substitution

When one stays in a hospital for medical treatment, coming into contact with tap water is unavoidable. From showering, brushing one's teeth, to taking an ice cube – tap water is everywhere in our daily routines. The notion of water as a vehicle for disease was not considered by hospitals until evidence began to surface of outbreaks linked to waterborne illnesses [16–19]. In our own experience at Children's National, T-cell-deficient patients experience a greater risk of developing nontuberculous mycobacterial infection after exposure to tap water during bathing and daily activities [20]. Strategies to mitigate these opportunistic infections include substituting tap water with distilled or sterile water for daily use and by maintaining a clean water system throughout the institution.

The CDC has estimated that four in five problems leading to US healthcare-associated outbreaks could be prevented with effective water management. When a water disinfection system in a building fails, such as by water not flowing properly, substandard disinfectant levels, or the presence of "deadlegs" (stagnant water), microbes that can be naturally found in bodies of water proliferate rapidly [21]. The higher the bacterial load in the water, the higher the likelihood that bacteria enter and infect a patient during contact. When a patient lacks a full immune system to defend the body, infections such as Legionnaires' disease can occur. Legionnaires' disease is a serious and deadly lung infection that kills 25% of those who contract the disease in a healthcare facility. Legionnaires' is caused by breathing in or aspirating small water droplets containing a pathogenic type of *Legionella* bacteria [22]. Among people who reported a site of exposure to Legionnaires' disease, 76% identified a healthcare facility as their exposure location [23]. To help building owners reduce the risk of *Legionella* growth and transmission, guidelines and standards have been developed by several agencies and professional groups [21]. *Legionella* water management programs are now an industry standard for large buildings in the United States (ASHRAE 188: Legionellosis: Risk Management for Building Water Systems June 26, 2015. ASHRAE: Atlanta) [23]. Hospitals are obligated to comply with the standard and to maintain a healthy water delivery system in the institution.

Engineering Control and Administrative Control

During infectious disease pandemics, such as influenza, COVID-19, and the Ebola virus, elimination (physically removing the hazard) and substitution (replacing the hazard) are not typically options. In these instances, engineering (isolating people from hazard) and administrative (changing the way people work) controls must be enforced to reduce and avoid exposure to these contagious illnesses. Prompt detection and effective triage and isolation of potentially infectious patients are essential to prevent unnecessary exposures among patients, healthcare providers, and visitors at the facility.

Beginning in late 2019, humans have confronted unprecedented challenges raised by the novel coronavirus – the SARS-COV-2 pandemic, more commonly known as COVID-19. The virus has all of the traits needed to cause a pandemic. It can spread quickly through respiratory droplets or aerosol among humans, and, as a novel disease, there is no natural immunity or vaccine to prevent infection and no effective therapy to treat infected patients. Hospitals must stay in operation and be ready to care for patients infected with COVID-19, while effective infection prevention and control strategies must be deployed to prevent the transmission of this virus from patients to staff and vice versa. Failure to control the spread of an infectious disease like COVID-19 in a hospital is reflected by hospital-onset infection among patient and occupational acquisition of the disease among staff.

In the context of engineering control, combating COVID-19 in the hospital starts with early identification and early isolation. Staff members actively reach out to families and patients before their scheduled visit to identify patients with signs and symptoms consistent with COVID-19 infection and proactively coordinate patients' visits, so that potential patients can be promptly isolated upon entering the hospital. With knowledge of a patient's infectious status, staff can take precautions during their patient interactions. When these preventive measures work in concert, safe care can be delivered to a patient without jeopardizing staff safety and the safety of other individuals.

When an infectious disease circulates in communities, healthcare workers are not immune to being infected and can even become a source of spread to patients and other coworkers. Thus, altering the way that staff work is prudent to reduce risks of spread. Taking advantage of our interconnectedness with the Internet, society, including the healthcare industry, has quickly adopted telemedicine, teleworking, virtual meetings, and other innovative communication methods and mitigated virus transmission risk associated with crowded spaces and contact with the sick. With employer commitment and employee buy-in, the consistent use of administrative control can effectively interrupt disease transmission in workplaces.

Personal Protective Equipment (PPE)

The duties of healthcare workers call on them to provide hands-on care to patients with known and unknown infectious diseases. Without knowing a patient's infectious disease status, PPE offers instant protection and must be included in the suite of strategies to protect personnel.

PPE, as defined by the Occupational Safety and Health Administration (OSHA) (an American governmental body that issues regulations for workplace health and safety) is any "specialized clothing or equipment worn by an employee for protection against infectious materials." The use of PPE in healthcare settings is required by the OSHA to protect healthcare personnel from exposure to bloodborne pathogens and other potentially infectious diseases. Hospitals, as employers, must provide appropriate PPE and ensure proper management and disposition of PPE after use. The CDC issues recommendations for when and what PPE should be used to prevent exposure to infectious diseases, and the Food and Drug Administration establishes standards that qualify a PPE to be used in healthcare settings and in special environments such as operating rooms.

All the types of PPE listed in Table 7.1 can be used individually or concurrently to protect healthcare workers from exposures to infectious diseases by creating a barrier between the worker and infectious material. When used appropriately, PPE reduces contamination of staff hands and clothing, therefore reducing the risk of transmitting infectious agents, including multidrug-resistant organisms.

The effectiveness of PPE is determined by three factors. Firstly, the selection of proper PPE should be based on anticipation of

Table 7.1 Types of PPE in healthcare settings

Gloves: protect hands
Gowns/aprons: protect skin and/or clothing
Masks and respirators: protect mouth/nose
Respirators – protect the respiratory tract from infectious agents
Goggles: protect eyes
Face shields: protect face, mouth, nose, and eyes

exposure and the type of exposure (i.e. blood, respiratory secretion, urine, etc.) and the durability and appropriateness of the PPE for the task and fit for the user. Correct PPE offers healthcare workers safety, durability, and comfort. Secondly, employees must obtain proper training in safely donning and, more importantly, doffing PPE to avoid the cross-contamination of hands, clothing, and surrounding objects. Thirdly, deciding the proper PPE for patient interactions should be based upon clinical interactions with a patient and the patient's status of infectivity [24]. Ultimately, while hospitals make PPE available to healthcare workers, for their own health, healthcare workers must take the matter into their own hands by knowing when to use what type of PPE and how to use it correctly every time.

The Importance of Connecting the Dots: A Case Study

Successful infection prevention and control in a hospital arises from the successful integration of infection control practices into every provider's practice with every patient. As described above, many strategies, techniques, and protective gear are available as options for healthcare providers to choose for patient interactions. This case study is to illustrate the importance of applying infection control principles and practices that are tailored to an individual's care.

The patient is a teenage male who was admitted for cancer remission during the COVID-19 pandemic. On the day of his admission, he was tested for COVID-19 to determine the status of his infectious disease. Because COVID-19 has a prolonged incubation period and the possibility of false negatives, a single test is unable to rule out the possibility of COVID-19 infection. Accordingly, staff members utilized universal precaution by wearing a surgical mask and eye protection when entering the patient's room to prevent exposure to COVID-19. A central line was placed on the patient for the rapid delivery of critical medication and for reducing pain and discomfort from repeat intravenous injections.

As the patient's condition deteriorated, the patient experienced skin breakdown at multiple body sites, intra-abdominal bleeding, diarrhea, and mucositis. The gross discomfort and the pain were so overwhelming that the patient was unwilling to carry on their daily routine, including basic personal hygiene. Eight days after admission, the patient developed a bloodstream infection caused by *Pseudomonas aeruginosa*. Although the patient recovered from the infection, his infection reveals that infection control principles, the chain of infection, and the hierarchy of control are imperative in an episode like this.

His medical condition and subsequent treatment marked the patient as a susceptible host for infection. The insertion of a central line, together with skin breakdowns, created multiple portals that facilitated the entry of *Pseudomonas aeruginosa* into the patient's bloodstream. This condition was worsened when he refused daily hygiene in the setting of diarrhea and further increased the risk of *Pseudomonas aeruginosa* transmission. Despite the concurrently raging COVID-19 pandemic, the staff understood that patient care must be provided. As such, all staff wore proper PPE, including surgical masks and face shields, for their own health and the health of others.

In this case, opportunities to break the chain of infection are limited, given the patient's overall condition and that an endogenous process might have contributed to the translocation of the infectious agent to the patient's bloodstream. Nonetheless, with the information available, this patient's infection meets the definition of a central line-associated bloodstream infection. Taking a closer view of this incident, the care team subsequently emphasized to all caregivers the need to escalate concerns promptly. In this case, the patient's poor personal hygiene and poor skin conditions merited concern and increased precaution.

Every staff member in a hospital plays a role in preventing HAIs. When infection control strategies are applied correctly in everyday practice, they can stop the spread of infection and protect the safety of both patients and staff members. Not every HAI is preventable, but every HAI should only occur after all prevention efforts have been exhausted. *Infection prevention and control is in everyone's hands.*

References

1. Hanninen O, Farago M, Monos E. Semmelweis' discovery and its Finnish follow-up. Acta Physiol Hung. 2003;90(2):83–95.
2. Miranda CM, Navarrete TL. Semmelweis and his outstanding contribution to medicine: washing hands saves lives. Rev Chil Infectol. 2008;25(1):54–7.
3. Allegranzi B, Storr J, Dziekan G, Leotsakos A, Donaldson L, Pittet D. The first global patient safety challenge "clean care is safer care": from launch to current progress and achievements. J Hosp Infect. 2007;65(Suppl 2):115–23.
4. Wise RI, Ossman EA, Littlefield DR. Personal reflections on nosocomial staphylococcal infections and the development of hospital surveillance. Rev Infect Dis. 1989;11(6):1005–19.
5. Services USDoHaH. Principles of epidemiology in public health practice: an introduction to applied epidemiology and biostatistics. Atlanta: U.S. Department of Health and Human Services, Centers for Disease Control and Prevention (CDC), Office of Workforce and Career Development; 2012.
6. See I, Freifeld AG, Causative Organisms MSS. Associated antimicrobial resistance in healthcare-associated, central line-associated bloodstream infections from oncology settings, 2009–2012. Clin Infect Dis. 2016;62(10):1203–9.
7. Green VW. Surgery, sterilization and sterility. J Healthc Mater Manage. 1993;11(2):46, 8–52.
8. Jarvis WR. Nosocomial outbreaks: the Centers for Disease Control's Hospital Infections Program experience, 1980–1990. Epidemiology Branch, Hospital Infections Program. Am J Med. 1991;91(3B):101S–6S.

9. Higa JT, Gluck M, Ross AS. Duodenoscope-associated bacterial infections: a review and update. Curr Treat Options Gastroenterol. 2016;14(2):185–93.
10. Kwok K, Chang J, Lo S, Giap A, Lim B, Wu B. A novel adjunctive cleansing method to reduce colony-forming units on duodenoscopes. Endosc Int Open. 2016;4(11):E1178–E82.
11. Rutala WA, Weber DJ. Outbreaks of carbapenem-resistant enterobacteriaceae infections associated with duodenoscopes: what can we do to prevent infections? Am J Infect Control. 2016;44(5 Suppl):e47–51.
12. Douce RW, Zurita J, Sanchez O, Cardenas Aldaz P. Investigation of an outbreak of central venous catheter-associated bloodstream infection due to contaminated water. Infect Control Hosp Epidemiol. 2008;29(4):364–6.
13. Kimura AC, Calvet H, Higa JI, Pitt H, Frank C, Padilla G, et al. Outbreak of Ralstonia pickettii bacteremia in a neonatal intensive care unit. Pediatr Infect Dis J. 2005;24(12):1099–103.
14. Moreira BM, Leobons MB, Pellegrino FL, Santos M, Teixeira LM, de Andrade Marques E, et al. Ralstonia pickettii and *Burkholderia cepacia* complex bloodstream infections related to infusion of contaminated water for injection. J Hosp Infect. 2005;60(1):51–5.
15. Romero-Gomez MP, Quiles-Melero MI, Pena Garcia P, Gutierrez Altes A, Garcia de Miguel MA, Jimenez C, et al. Outbreak of *Burkholderia cepacia* bacteremia caused by contaminated chlorhexidine in a hemodialysis unit. Infect Control Hosp Epidemiol. 2008;29(4):377–8.
16. Garvey MI, Wilkinson MAC, Holden KL, Martin T, Parkes J, Holden E. Tap out: reducing waterborne *Pseudomonas aeruginosa* transmission in an intensive care unit. J Hosp Infect. 2019;102(1):75–81.
17. Moffa M, Guo W, Li T, Cronk R, Abebe LS, Bartram J. A systematic review of nosocomial waterborne infections in neonates and mothers. Int J Hyg Environ Health. 2017;220(8):1199–206.
18. Safiri S, Ayubi E. *Pseudomonas aeruginosa* outbreak in a neonatal intensive care unit attributed to hospital tap water: methodological and statistical issues to avoid misinterpretation. Infect Control Hosp Epidemiol. 2017;38(9):1126–7.
19. Umezawa K, Asai S, Ohshima T, Iwashita H, Ohashi M, Sasaki M, et al. Outbreak of drug-resistant Acinetobacter baumannii ST219 caused by oral care using tap water from contaminated hand hygiene sinks as a reservoir. Am J Infect Control. 2015;43(11):1249–51.
20. Davila Saldana BJ, Keller M, Hanisch BR, Song X. Tap water: a possible source of nontuberculous mycobacterial infection in patients with T cell deficiency. Am J Infect Control. 2019;47(7):834–6.
21. NIOSH. In: Burton N, Afanuh S, editors. Preventing occupational exposure to Legionella. Cincinnati: U.S. Department of Health and Human Services, Centers for Disease Control and Prevention, National Institute for Occupational Safety and Health, DHHS (NIOSH) Publication No. 2019-131; 2019. https://doi.org/10.26616/NIOSHPUB20191312019.

22. CDC. Signs and symptoms: Legionnaires' disease 2018. Available from: https://www.cdc.gov/legionella/about/signs-symptoms.html
23. CDC. Developing a water management program to reduce Legionella growth and spread in buildings: a practical guide to implementing industry standards. Atlanta: U.S. Department of Health and Human Services, Centers for Disease Control and Prevention; 2017. https://www.cdc.gov/legionella/downloads/toolkit.pdf
24. CDC. Guidance for the selection and use of personal protective equipment (PPE) in healthcare settings 2004. Available from: https://www.cdc.gov/hai/pdfs/ppe/ppeslides6-29-04.pdf

Technology and Health Care Improvement

8

Jessica Herstek and Eric Shelov

Health information technology (IT) encompasses multiple overlapping electronic hardware and software systems that enable clinical services across health care settings today. Federal inventive programs propelled the adoption of electronic health records (EHRs) and other medical software systems in a majority of hospitals and clinics over the past decade. Much focus during this time was on implementation, getting up and running on electronic equivalents of preexisting paper processes. While many types of errors and inefficiencies have been eliminated in this phase of expanding use, new risks and unintended consequences have emerged. Clinicians, informaticists, and IT developers, engineers, and companies are now partnering as health IT evolves to maximize its potential to support safer and high-quality health care for patients and decreased burden and frustration for clinicians.

J. Herstek (✉)
Department of Pediatrics, The George Washington University School of Medicine and Health Sciences, Children's National Hospital, Washington, DC, USA
e-mail: jherstek@childrensnational.org

E. Shelov
Department of Biomedical & Health Informatics, Division of General Pediatrics, Perelman School of Medicine, University of Pennsylvania, Children's Hospital of Philadelphia, Philadelphia, PA, USA
e-mail: shelov@chop.edu

R. Roberts-Turner, R. K. Shah (eds.), *Pocket Guide to Quality Improvement in Healthcare*,
https://doi.org/10.1007/978-3-030-70780-4_8

The Next Phase

Gone are the days when IT was just another department in the fluorescent-lit basement of a hospital or office building. Health IT systems now underpin every clinical care activity, from the way doctors and nurses communicate and document care to the automated tools that are intended to add layers of safety to inherently risky and complex processes and procedures. EHRs are the foundational systems that capture the bulk of clinical data created by the minute and hour in the course of care, though health IT today comprises a multitude of parallel interfaced devices and systems.

Even the most basic EHRs were implemented in only around 10% of hospitals in 2009, the year that the federal HITECH Act was passed to incentivize adoption, but was approaching 100% a decade later [1]. Given the transformational potential of this trend, this has been a phenomenal accomplishment. We understand intuitively now the safety of legible prescriptions, the convenience of electronic communication, and the value of instant access to information for both patients and health care professionals. But what was not broadly appreciated until more recently was the double-edged sword that digitization and automation represent.

EHRs are plagued by a litany of complaints from health care workers and patients alike. Poor usability, cognitive overload, alert fatigue, and automation complacency are examples of health hazards that technology has introduced. Counterintuitive user interfaces stem from a lack of user-centered design, where clinicians have input on engineering decisions early in the project to make the system work best for them. Propagation of information overload leads to dangerous phenomena such as alert fatigue, where clinicians become conditioned to ignore meaningless yet interruptive signals from the system, at the risk of missing actual critical signals. Even when systems are perceived as highly reliable, an overreliance on technology can result in automation bias and operator complacency, an inappropriate degree of trust in the system over human input or common sense. Today's EHRs and related health IT products offer innumerable advantages over legacy systems and have been an integral part of improving patient safety. Yet even as they have addressed many inherently unsafe processes by digitizing handwritten medical records, electronic systems introduce these and other new safety risks into health care.

Health IT systems can and should be leveraged as the robust safety and quality improvement tools they are. But no matter how much time, effort, and money are spent on implementation, failure to recognize that no electronic or automated system is intrinsically, infallibly safe can have startling consequences.

In Error

A teenaged boy holds a cup of pills in his hand. He places a pill in his mouth, swallows, and takes another. Then another and another. Then a handful at a time. He doesn't stop until he has swallowed 39 pills.

He is not alone. He is with a young woman who watches him closely. She doesn't leave until she sees that he took all 39 pills. Doctor's orders.

The woman is his nurse. The boy is in the hospital. His mother is nearby, in another room with his younger brother, who is also sick in the hospital on this particular night. The pill is an antibiotic the boy takes every day at home to prevent infections. He has a genetic condition that affects his immune system, and the pill usually helps keep him out of the hospital. At home he takes a single pill twice a day, every day. He was not admitted to the hospital for an infection this time – the pill had been doing its job. He was there for a routine procedure.

Later that night, the boy notices numbness and tingling all over his body. Then, after texting with a friend, he suddenly screams for his mother. His body goes stiff, limbs shaking, jaw clenched, and back arched against the hospital bed. His breathing stops. A "code blue" is called. He survives the seizure but is transferred to the intensive care unit, where he will have to remain in the hospital much longer than planned.

The 39 pills were an unintentional overdose ordered by the resident physician, approved by the pediatric pharmacist, handed over by the bedside nurse, and dutifully taken by the boy. Between each of these – by all accounts – competent and caring health care professionals and the patient lay an elaborate electronic safety system, meant to remove all the points at which such errors could transpire. This case occurred at a prestigious academic medical center, within reach of Silicon Valley, that had invested heavily in technology to further patient safety [2]. Hundreds of millions of dollars in equipment and staff time spent training and typing and clicking and scanning conspired to create a nonsensical medication error.

Necessary But Not Sufficient

This type of massive overdose would almost certainly have not occurred in the era before widespread use of health IT systems. The particular circumstances that allowed the error to occur stemmed directly from the multiple layers of technology in place, as detailed by Dr. Robert Wachter in his examination of this case in his book, "The Digital Doctor: Hope, Hype, and Harm at the Dawn of Medicine's Computer Age" [2]. The advent of technology in health care was a necessary surge forward in patient safety, but clearly, the use of high-tech tools is not sufficient to prevent harm to patients nor adequate to support clinicians in their work.

Many doctors practicing today trained in an era of handwritten notes, hand-signed orders, and scribbled prescriptions. In this world, a doctor 24 hours in to a 30-plus-hour shift could hastily scrawl an incomplete order for a medication on a piece of paper, which was then faxed to the pharmacy, yielding faint scratchings that translated to a drug or dosing error. Pharmacy staff could grab the wrong bottle off the shelf before counting out pills and sending them to the unit. A nurse could give a dose intended for an obese adult patient to the small child down the hall instead. These flagrant errors all could have happened and did with frightening regularity. We can now prevent these in part with the installation of complex and expensive technology meant to keep patients safe, yet an unprecedented overdose still reached a patient in the current era. These types of errors continue to occur with regularity across health care settings. Implementation and optimization of EHRs and related systems are a necessary but not sufficient component of any patient safety program.

A joint investigation conducted by Kaiser Health News and Fortune magazine reviewed the federal government's decade-long, 36-billion-dollar incentive program to convert medical records from paper to electronic. This conversion promised freedom from all the limitations, inefficiencies, and well-documented safety issues in previous decades that could be traced back to reams of paper. In the scathing review, the reporters cataloged medicolegal cases implicating EHRs. Cases are detailed of missed or delayed diagnoses due to EHR errors with catastrophic consequences. The EHR vendors in these cases blamed clients for user error, inadequate training, or improper setup of their systems. Hospitals blamed EHR companies for poor visual layout and unintuitive user design. "It can be hard to tell where human error begins and the technological shortcomings end" [3]. Physicians and nurses in general don't have any better views of EHRs. Surgeon and writer Atul Gawande penned an article about EHRs in 2018 in The New Yorker called "Why Doctors Hate Their Computers," in which he notes the frustrations, limitations, and information overload many clinicians experience working with current systems [4].

There is no question that electronic systems save lives, but thoughtful design, careful implementation, and continuous quality improvement are required to prevent or mitigate unintended consequences and novel error types, too.

Closing Loops

The process of ordering medications in any hospital is fraught with potential for harm. Whether paper or electronic, it involves dozens of steps. Each step represents an opportunity for error, but also an opportunity for assistance from technology. Medication processes that can be facilitated by EHRs and related systems, and are recommended by the federal government, include computerized provider order entry, clinical decision support, and bar-coded medication administration systems [5, 6]. Primarily over the last decade, hospitals spent tens or even hundreds of millions of dollars to purchase and implement computerized provider order entry systems. These systems finally eliminated the risk of misinterpretation of a doctor's handwriting, loss of paper order sheets, or poor fax transmission quality to the pharmacy leading to wrong drug or dose errors, among a myriad of other well-documented issues. Additionally, rather than starting with a blank sheet of paper, and consulting a pocket reference or other external dosing guide, an ordering provider can be presented with appropriately calibrated choices with built-in guidance specific to that patient and clinical scenario in order to support their decision-making. This system of computerized knowledge is referred to as clinical decision support. A third component towards safer, "closed-loop" medication processes entails bar-coded medication administration tools. With these tools, nurses at the patient bedside can scan bar codes or other machine-readable tags imprinted on medication packaging and an identification bracelet on the patient, prior to administering the drug. The system cross-checks the patient and drug with the original medication ordered by the physician in the EHR. The final step confirms that the correct drug was delivered and is administered to the intended patient.

In addition to a robust EHR with computerized provider order entry, clinical decision support, and bar-coded medication administration modules, the hospital where this massive overdose occurred had also spent millions of dollars on a pharmacy robot to select, dispense, and deliver routine medications. This investment freed the pharmacy staff to focus on more nuanced work that requires human attention. The combination of these systems embedded in the EHR, the pharmacy robot, and the bar-coded medication administration process were meant to prevent errors at each of the major inflection points in medication ordering, dispensing, and administration. In other words, this hospital had put in place all the latest recommended technology systems to provide closed-loop medication administration, starting from correct order entry and ending with giving the right medication to the right patient.

Despite all these high-tech safety systems, errors are still widely reported. An identification bracelet can be lost or placed on the wrong patient, a pharmacist or manufacturer can mislabel a medication bag or vial. A nurse can – and sometimes must – find a workaround to administer a fluid or medication to the patient without delay when the bar code scanner is not connecting to the system via Bluetooth. All the issues with electronic systems we all run into in our own daily lives happen with health IT, too. Wires get unplugged, batteries run out, mobile units go missing, systems freeze, and a wireless pairing fails. Yet the delivery of health care must proceed, with or without these safety supports in place.

So what went wrong in this case? There was in fact no spectacular technologic failure, but a combination of issues with people, process, and technology that culminated in the dozens of pills reaching the patient. The introduction of each new layer of safety comes with both benefits and risks. In fact, technology can create novel and sometimes unanticipated sources of error. In this case, poor usability, alert fatigue, and automation bias were complicit. These phenomena are essential for quality and safety teams to understand, as they must be considered when reviewing safety incidents involving health IT systems, as well as when leveraging health IT to address patient safety issues or quality improvement efforts. The introduction of EHR systems designed, historically, by non-clinicians has led to disastrous examples of the limits of technology to eliminate errors altogether. As with any complex, high-risk, and evolving system, a continuous quality improvement approach should be taken to implementing and maintaining health IT systems, as the hardware and software as well as user training and cultural norms will inevitably change over time.

Calibrating Trust

The doctor who ordered the overdose had actually entered the order correctly in the computer system earlier that day. But because the dose calculator was overly precise, there was a rounding issue. And because there was a rounding issue, the reviewing pharmacist, following hospital policy, called the doctor back to reenter the correct, rounded dose. This time, the doctor entered the order a slightly different way, with little visual indication of a mistaken unit of measure. The ease with which this doctor committed an extreme prescribing error on a commonly used medication in the EHR can be blamed on poor usability of the order interface. A well-designed user interface can prevent or at least deter simple mistakes in order entry. After signing the incorrect order, she did, however, receive a pop-up alert warning of the overdose, as did the pharmacist. They both clicked habitually through these warnings, due to the frequency of such alerts that were often meaningless. This is attributable to alert or notification fatigue – the concept that the quantity, design, and calibration of alerts in any system can dramatically alter cognitive processing and response to the information being presented. Based on their past experiences with unhelpful alerts, both the doctor and the pharmacist were unintentionally trained to mistrust the EHR's alerts, even though in this case it was giving them critical feedback on their actions.

Clearly, all the built-in knowledge embedded in the EHR can backfire, manifesting as alert fatigue among clinicians, with real consequences on patient safety and clinician satisfaction. Articles in the medical literature describe techniques to address alert fatigue and poor usability of EHRs. In one paper, researchers from Harvard Medical School created an algorithm to use "cranky comments" that doctors typed in responses to pop-up alerts in the EHR to detect programming errors [7]. The prestigious New England Journal of Medicine published a hospital system's popular EHR improvement campaign titled "Getting Rid of Stupid Stuff," detailing their use of clinician input to address serious problems such as alert fatigue [8]. The phenomenon of alert fatigue is now so well-recognized that it is called out in the nonprofit ECRI Institute's annual report of Top 10 Health Technology Hazards [9].

To mitigate this risk, the process of designing alerts and other electronic tools can be improved by focusing on usability. Usability refers to the design of the user interface of a system, whether a button on a car dashboard or in a hospital's EHR. Products or systems with good usability are intuitive, not requiring hours or days of training, to start using and use correctly. They are efficient, not engendering frustration by requiring multiple clicks or interruptions that are of low value or yield to the user. For EHRs, usability addresses how well the system helps health care workers complete their tasks and how well its user interface balances efficiency and safety by minimizing human error. This relates to both broad functionality and the detailed design of visual layout. The risk of unintentional selection of the wrong item, or of missing an important system prompt, is directly affected by design choices. Errors can stem from displaying too much information, requiring extensive scrolling, grouping items too close together, or using too small a font. One factor known to lead to poor usability is a lack of user-centered design or appreciation for the criticality of the human-computer interface.

Improving the usability of EHRs is not just an imperative to mitigate clinician frustration but also for patient safety. Many EHR vendors now employ human factors engineers and usability experts and leverage user-centered design methods that were often absent from earlier iterations of current EHR systems. Clinicians, too, have responded to the clear need to filter design and decision-making through the lens of usability. In fact, the need is so great that an entirely new specialty of medicine was created to train and certify physicians to work in this area. Clinical informatics became an official subspecialty of the American Board of Preventive Medicine in 2013 – the same year the boy described above was given an extreme overdose both despite, and because of, health IT systems in place. Physicians, nurses, and other health care professionals who work in informatics act as crucial partners with frontline clinicians, software engineers who design the systems, and hospital IT staff who are tasked with configuring and customizing these systems. Inclusion of informatics-trained clinicians in improvement projects can help the project team select and design appropriate EHR interventions, as well as take advantage of electronic systems to measure change.

Making the Right Thing Easy

Most fundamentally, the goal of clinical decision support is to present information to a clinician in real time and expect that they take action of some kind. At first pass this may seem straightforward, but there are many elements to be considered when developing decision support, and the consequences of not being thoughtful in this development can be significant. Medicine is hardly the first industry with technology attempting to assist in its productivity, and over the years clinical informaticists have learned valuable lessons and started to define and refine best practices. Perhaps the most important lesson learned in the health IT field is that out-of-the-box technology by itself is unlikely to solve a clinical problem. Rather, for effective solutions to be deployed, significant analysis of the problem at hand and the workflow involved are critical prerequisites to determine how best to incorporate technology tools like clinical decision support.

Relatively early in the field of clinical informatics, a group of researchers defined the "Ten Commandments" for successful clinical decision support [10]. These best practices include redirecting as opposed to stopping the user, recognizing the importance of speed in clinical work, and paying careful attention to workflow. Although this workflow analysis requires an investment of resources, it is nearly always worth the effort when the clinical decision support tool is built. Of note, there are excellent quality improvement tools that can play a vital role in this kind of analysis. Techniques such as driver diagrams and swimlane analysis can help represent the details of complex workflows that are needed before beginning the process of proper decision support development.

An additional framework that has evolved in the informatics literature is the concept of the "Five Rights" of clinical decision support [11]. The rights include the following:

- *Right information*: Evidence- or consensus-based, suitable to guide action.
- *Right person*: Including all members of the care team. Increasingly with electronic patient portals, this may also include patients and families.
- *Right time*: At the time of decision-making and desired action.

- *Right channel*: These may include both digital channels, such as the EHR, and non-digital such as signs at the bedside.
- *Right format*: Once a channel is determined, the right tool must be used, for example, an order set versus an alert.

These principles are helpful when considering a specific decision support tool, but during the design phase, it may be more practical to consider a question-oriented format. In the ideal scenario, standard tools are first used to analyze a problem, complete a workflow analysis, and identify necessary behavior changes. At that point, a series of questions can help to determine the right decision support approach. Who is the person or role that needs to change their behavior? What information do they need? When do they need it? What action do we expect them to take? These questions are the five rights of clinical decision support framed in a question-oriented format.

By answering these questions before committing to a particular approach in the EHR, quality improvement teams have a much better chance of choosing the right tool as opposed to one that is familiar but is poorly aligned with workflow. Unfortunately, this kind of analysis has historically not taken place when clinical teams design decision support. Instead, they are often developed quickly, in a reactive manner, jumping to common but blunt tools like pop-up alerts. Alerts developed in this manner tend to be ineffective in the long run, as the target audience quickly becomes accustomed to the alert's presence if it is not properly calibrated. Worse still, they propagate the sense that the EHR system is poorly designed, inefficient, and frustrating for busy frontline clinicians and, as we have seen, can lead to patient harm rather than prevent it as intended.

Clinical decision support systems can both save physicians clicks and time and steer them toward desirable choices or away from risky or otherwise undesirable prescribing behaviors. Their actions can even be forced, depending on how restrictive the design of the clinical decision support tool is. Linking in access to vast databases can support clinical decision-making by having the computer tap into knowledge resources and providing, for example, cross-checks on standard dose ranges, drug interactions with other medications, or allergies that may otherwise go unnoticed. More advanced displays provide the physician with access to the latest clinical guidelines for their patient's condition or, better yet, implement it as the default pathway so that it requires extra effort and attention on the part of the physician to deviate from the standard of care. This is sometimes appropriate, and physicians may require and desire flexibility to customize patient care at their discretion. Often, however, patient safety and quality of care benefit from standardization where such approaches exist. In many cases, this can be readily accomplished with built-in templates of orders, termed order sets, which can help standardize care and promote education of providers at the same time. Order sets are perhaps the most frequently used decision support tool employed to support quality improvement efforts, with every modern EHR supporting this functionality in one way or another.

Order sets can most fundamentally be thought of as a collection of provider orders commonly grouped together to facilitate entry. On the less sophisticated side, an order set may simply be a reference for commonly used tests or medications for a particular scenario or clinical condition, such as treating an asthma attack or managing postoperative pain. In more sophisticated forms, order sets can represent a clinical pathway, algorithm, or decision tree with highly prescriptive guidance through each anticipated phase of care. Additional features provided by many EHRs include default selection of particular orders to encourage or even mandate their inclusion, nested groups of orders where a single selection leads to a cascade of additional selections, and the ability to hide or show orders based on available data about that particular patient, such as age and gender. Logic can be built in, for example, to automatically add a pregnancy test when indicated for female patients in an appropriate age range, but not display at all for male patients. This ensures extra protections for pregnant patients while decreasing the chances that a provider inadvertently orders the test when not applicable.

In the overdose case reviewed above, the ordering physician had to type in a specific numeric dose for the patient's home medication, leaving vulnerable several variables in each order, including unit of measure, intended strength, and formulation. Because this particular drug came in tablet form, with very standardized dosing across almost all patients, forcing the doctor to enter these details anew every time adds unnecessary steps to the ordering process and increases opportunity for error. If the order fields for that medication had been pre-filled out to include only the numeric dose available per pill, she would have had less clicks to enter and less chance of doing it incorrectly. Better still, she could have selected the correct choice for that patient automatically from within an order set dedicated to, for example, patients with compromised immune systems who often take this medication every day. Moreover, modern EHRs can filter options being displayed, so in this case the system "knew" the patient was an adolescent and therefore could have predicted that he would take the standard adult dose of that medication. The default choice displayed to the doctor, such as a pre-checked dose, usually represents the path of least resistance. In other words, the easiest or most obvious available action on any view presented to the provider should contain the most common or correct option, raising the likelihood of a busy, stressed, distracted, or inexperienced provider entering a safe order. To maximize the benefits of order sets, careful consideration must be given to align the order set with the clinical decision-making process in an algorithm or pathway. The ease and effectiveness with which a clinical guideline can be translated into meaningful decision support will depend on its design and language. If a guideline or clinical pathway is full of ambiguity and points of indecision, it will be challenging to create an order set that clinicians find useful and are therefore willing to use [12].

There are many success stories of order sets that resulted in significant improvements in clinical care when built on the foundation of a thoughtful clinical pathway. This is facilitated by considering a pathway as a clinical decision tree, with the information presented at moments of decision to guide the clinician in the right direction for the patient. Order sets can be created to reflect this very same structure, with key data from the patient and pertinent reference information included right at the point of decision-making in the workflow. The provider then has all the information needed to make the correct or best decision for that patient. This approach has been taken to decrease the use of popular but overly expensive drugs or tests, such as an intravenous form of the common fever medicine acetaminophen in children who can just as easily take it by mouth, or to make sure physicians order a blood test for certain patients prior to starting antibiotics. That test being ordered at the proper time provides crucial information to the medical team that cannot be obtained once antibiotics have been started. The order set prompts the physician to include it every time, instead of relying on them to remember to add it manually and risk missing a diagnosis that can help tailor the subsequent treatment plan.

On the other hand, there are also many cautionary tales where order sets do not align with a particular clinical pathway and result in unintended consequences. For example, a team designing a pathway may want to discourage the use of a particular test for a certain condition, due to expense, harm, or other downstream effects. In children who develop a common and uncomplicated respiratory infection, ordering a chest X-ray is often unnecessary to safely diagnosis and treat the condition. The X-ray not only adds cost to the parents' health care expenses but exposes the child to radiation without direct benefit and, further, could lead to overdiagnosis of otherwise benign conditions with a cascade of subsequent added costs, risks, and worries. The obvious approach may be to simply not include that X-ray order in an order set used for this type of patient. While this may certainly achieve some gains, it is likely some providers will go outside the order set to find the X-ray order and order it anyway. These providers would then deem that order set not useful since it does not contain all the orders they are accustomed to using. The next time they see a similar patient, they are less likely to use the order set and thereby miss out on the other benefits of streamlined and standardized care driven by evidence-based electronic pathways. One possible approach to prevent this from happening could be to actually include the X-ray order in the order set but display specific instructions or links to evidence-based resources supporting the rationale behind limiting its use. This serves not only to discourage inappropriate use of the study, but it also provides relevant education and real-time feedback to the provider who has been in the habit of using such a test indiscriminately.

The Signal and the Noise

In addition to well-designed orders and order sets, one of the other most common interventions that can support quality improvement work is an electronic alert. Alerts can be broadly defined as an automated flag or indicator meant to get the user's attention. They come in countless forms and representations such as icons, banners, or pop-up windows with text, figures, and buttons that may need to be clicked to bypass the alert and return to the original workflow. Alerts are a tool fraught with challenges in the EHR. While they hold much promise to change behavior, their overuse has led to significant frustration and unintended, potentially fatal, consequences in the EHR [13]. Health care is not alone in struggling with how to best deploy alerts. Aerospace and nuclear power industries have also learned hard lessons on the benefits and unintended consequences of alert design, particularly those that interrupt the thoughts and actions of a doctor, pilot, or other professional performing high-risk work. These streams constitute workflow, and its analysis is integral to designing useful alerts.

A well-designed alert constitutes a critical signal from the system to the clinician of a scenario or action with potentially dire consequences. When that signal is sent to the wrong person, at the wrong time, or through the wrong channel, it can be lost in the noise of all the other, less important alerts. Ideally, the EHR should serve as a trusted advisor to clinicians, delivering timely guidance and relevant suggestions integrated smoothly within their workflow. Electronic alerts have historically taken a more adversarial tone with clinicians, but today clinical informatics professionals and EHR vendors are actively trying to course-correct, to everyone's benefit.

Alerts have several characteristics to consider before use. They can be proactive, guiding clinicians towards the right thing, or reactive, stopping them when they have potentially done the wrong thing. They can be made to be intentionally interruptive, commonly in the form of a separate window popping up in a workflow, as opposed to non-interruptive, such as a banner or flag that can be acknowledged at their convenience without interruption. Whenever possible, decision support should be proactive and non-interruptive, striving to make the right thing easy rather than penalizing the clinician for having done the wrong thing.

The consequences of poor alert design and implementation are important to recognize. Alert fatigue emerges when clinicians must bypass numerous insignificant or irrelevant alerts in the course of their usual work and then miss or unintentionally override those few alerts that may be most important. Alerts that contain incorrect or misleading information also cause harm when clinicians, accustomed to relying on alerts to catch errors, act on false information without independent verification. This is an example of automation bias, which increases the more accurate any clinical decision support system is. Well-designed alerts and other clinical decision support can decrease harm overall to patients, but clinicians should be educated on automation bias. Clinicians must remain vigilant in environments with high automation and should be trained to maintain a culture of safety and use clinical judgment in conjunction with clinical decision support systems. In the case of ordering medications in a computerized prescribing system, for example, prescribers should consider the decision support system a secondary, independent check on the dose or indication for a medication [14].

Before selecting an EHR alert as an intervention for a quality improvement project, consider the test characteristics, such as how often it is right and how often it may fire inappropriately. Consider the design, from use of color to font size to wording, and consider the workflow, where in the many cognitive and physical steps the optimal timing is for the alert to fire. The severity of the clinical scenario should dictate how forceful the alert is, distinguishing life-threatening situations from best practice or cost-associated concerns, and the action(s) required of the clinician to either accept, override, or bypass the warning. The text of the alert should be designed in collaboration with the frontline clinicians who are the intended recipient of that contextual information, alongside informatics-trained clinicians when available, rather than by the quality improvement or IT teams independently – this is an example of the application of user-centered design. This approach helps achieve the desired goals of high usability and avoidance of unintended consequences. Even though changes can and should be made after go-live, the risks of inadequate initial design are high. In addition to immediate harm from use in the live patient environment, busy clinicians may get accustomed to the first impression made by a poorly performing alert, and their minds are not easily changed even if it is subsequently improved.

Even using good design principles, following up on the utility of the alert in the live environment remains as important as the initial design. The evidence is growing that clinical decision support testing can and should be performed "silently," or more accurately, invisibly, in live EHR systems with real patient data and fully functional interfaces, instead of in an isolated test environment as has been done traditionally. The results of this testing can thereby better inform the alert criteria and design. The criteria can be refined and improved based on actual patient data rather than scripted testing scenarios. Once alert criteria have been optimized, the final test characteristics should inform elements including the degree of interruption and the language displayed to the clinician. Methods of quantifying alert performance have improved and can facilitate ongoing improvement cycles.

In the previous overdose example, both the physician and the pharmacist received a number of pop-up alerts in the process of ordering and approving the medication. The alerts were reactive, occurring after the erroneous order had already been signed, and interruptive, triggering the instinctive behavior to click through the screens as quickly as possible to resume patient care activities. Furthermore, there was little visual distinction between these critical – and correct – massive overdose alerts and innumerable other trivial alerts all staff received routinely through the usual course of care. This is evidence of lack of user-centered design and is the setting that gives rise to alert fatigue.

On the other hand, the nurse in this case had come to rely on the accuracy of the bar code scanning system. It emitted a reassuring audible and visual signal every time a medication was scanned successfully showing a match between patient, drug, and order, and no mismatch was detected in this case. That system had worked so well, in fact, that the nurse ignored common sense and her own gut feeling that the dose was off. This natural tendency to trust automated systems despite evidence to the contrary is a manifestation of automation bias. In the everyday use of health IT systems, it is important to instill in all clinicians a healthy skepticism, especially during high-risk activities such as medication processing. Regardless of how automated or reliable an electronic system is, human behavior matters. Growing overreliance on technology, or automation complacency, is human nature. Maintaining a culture of safety becomes even more important with advanced technologies and automation.

Making It Count

Any quality improvement effort requires measurement, and informatics-based interventions are no exception. Informatics interventions can be assessed by the impact on structure, process, and/or outcome, with the ultimate goal of improving clinical outcomes. Not every informatics project can or should measure clinical outcomes, for example, if a specific process has clearly demonstrated tight linkage to a clinical outcome in previous research. This is particularly relevant for very rare events that may not occur with enough frequency at an individual institution to effectively demonstrate change. Process measures in the field of informatics have some unique challenges, however. The determination of what to measure is not always straightforward. As with any improvement effort, a discussion of what will be measured must be part of the planning for the intervention. As described above, the goal of many informatics interventions in the EHR are to change provider behavior in some way, so choices of what to measure boil down to the critical element of the workflow. In the current state of overburdened EHR users, informaticists strive to measure passively, leveraging actions clinicians take in the routine care of patients without introducing additional clicks or steps solely for the purpose of tracking. Some of these measures can be relatively straightforward, while others require greater sophistication for quality improvement project teams to assemble and interpret.

Orders are perhaps the easiest discrete unit to measure from the EHR and are a very reliable indicator of changes to patient care. Implementation of a pneumonia pathway, for example, could measure specific antibiotic usage in a defined cohort and determine whether or not the pathway achieved a particular goal in standardizing care. Nonmedication orders, such as those for specific nursing or supportive care, can also serve as useful metrics, but one must keep in mind that unlike medications, these orders may not always precisely correlate with the intended action. One type of order is nurse communication orders, which serve as standing free text instructions to nursing staff. An order that simply instructs a bedside nurse to "Apply vascular access care bundle," for example, may not be the best process metric to determine whether or not the bundle was applied. Fortunately, there are other discrete data elements that can serve as process metrics. Flowsheet documentation, commonly used by nursing staff, is a reportable discrete data source. These charts indicating completion of bundle elements such as central line inspection, dressing changes, and flushes would be more clinically meaningful metrics and just as readily retrieved from the EHR database.

Other useful data, although somewhat more difficult to extract and interpret, to serve as process metrics include metadata (data about data), alert interaction, and documentation data. An example of metadata would be attributes of particular orders, such as time of day ordered (e.g., during morning rounds), or whether or not the user ordered it as a standalone order or as part of a specific order set. A team working to improve sepsis care may want to measure whether orders for antibiotics, blood tests, and intravenous fluids derived from a specific order set they designed to standardize sepsis care. Alert data may initially seem straightforward, simply looking at how often an alert appears and is either bypassed by the user, if this is permitted, or leads the user to change what they were doing, such as changing a drug dose after seeing an overdose alert. Considering the numerous ways non-interruptive alerts may appear, however, and the variable actions or responses a clinician can take subsequently, it becomes more challenging. Sophisticated alerts with complex criteria and multiple action options may be challenging to compare to one another. Nonetheless, an informatics team may still find value in tracking metrics of a specific alert over time. Even with relatively straightforward interruptive alerts such as allergy or dose alerts, override rates are not always an accurate measure of alert performance.

Clinical documentation is another potential source of metric data, but it is one that presents unique challenges. Historically, clinical documentation was non-discrete and highly narrative. With the introduction of the EHR, there has been a shift towards discrete documentation with elements like mandatory fields and checklists. While this has been helpful for data capture, many in the medical field have lamented the loss of the narrative, arguably the most important part of medical care, cognitive processes, and learning. As it stands currently, documentation is largely a mixture of discrete and non-discrete elements. While the ability of natural language processing tools to extract reportable data from narrative text has advanced significantly in recent years, it remains a tool largely beyond the reach of most medical systems and clinical quality improvement teams. Thus, when physician notes are the only source of truth in the EHR for a particular question, such as a patient-reported symptom or the physician's thought process and decision-making, a manual review of notes remains the only option to leverage this kind of data.

More recently, techniques have emerged to create clinical documentation templates that provide data on the author's thought process. For example, a note template for pneumonia can be designed to offer select choices of text, rather than prompting free text entry, depending on clinical considerations such as severity of presenting symptoms, choosing from a drop-down menu of "moderate" or "severe," or their management plan referencing consideration of pneumonia. In many cases, the choices clinicians make as they complete the template can be recorded and used as a project metric. Embedded note data elements could help a quality team track how often physicians considered a diagnosis of pneumonia when patients present with severe respiratory symptoms.

Finally, to support continuous quality improvement efforts regarding the safety and usability of the EHR itself, informatics and quality improvement teams can now measure how clinicians are interacting with the EHR software more directly. Built-in software can monitor the time spent in a particular section of the chart, determine whether or not specific data was reviewed, or track the number of clicks spent on particular tasks. Unfortunately, this data can be quite challenging to work with. Not all EHR vendors make this data available, and when they do, it can be difficult to interpret without a deep understanding of EHR database structures. Increasingly this kind of data is being studied by informatics researchers to address systemic safety concerns that include documentation burden and alert fatigue.

Onward

The past decade of experience has illustrated the power and pitfalls of health information technology to readily implement clinical decision support interventions, including well-designed orders, order sets, alerts, and other tools to prompt or prevent targeted provider actions. Quality improvement teams can implement and enforce change quickly and broadly. EHRs support the measurement of successes and failures to support rapid-cycle change and iterative progress. With the majority of health care systems, from small private practices to large hospital networks, now using EHRs and complementary technologies, we are entering a new phase of more advanced thinking to design, use, and improve these all-encompassing systems proactively. This shift to EHRs and accompanying technologies impacts almost every facet of patient safety and quality of care. We all must bear in mind the principles of usability, mitigation of alert fatigue, and education and training to counterbalance the tendency toward automation bias and automation complacency. Technology solutions will continue to mature. Our approach to building and interacting with these systems must evolve, too, to address errors old and new.

References

1. The Office of the National Coordinator for Health Information Technology. Health IT dashboard. https://dashboard.healthit.gov/quickstats/pages/FIG-Hospital-EHR-Adoption.php
2. Wachter R. The digital doctor: hope, hype, and harm at the dawn of medicine's computer age. New York: McGraw Hill; 2015.
3. Shulte F, Fortune FE. Death by 1,000 clicks: where electronic health records went wrong. Mar 18, 2019. https://fortune.com/longform/medical-records/
4. Gawande A. Why doctors hate their computers. The New Yorker Magazine. Nov 5, 2018. https://www.newyorker.com/magazine/2018/11/12/why-doctors-hate-their-computers
5. The Office of the National Coordinator for Health Information Technology. Health IT playbook. http://healthit.gov/playbook/quality-and-patient-safety/
6. Institute for Healthcare Improvement. Improve core processes for administering medications. http://www.ihi.org/resources/Pages/Changes/ImproveCoreProcessesforAdministeringMedications.aspx
7. Aaron S, McEvoy D, Ray S, Hickman TT, Wright A. Cranky comments: detecting clinical decision support malfunctions through free-text override reasons. J Am Med Inform Assoc. 2019;26(1):37–43. https://doi.org/10.1093/jamia/ocy139.
8. Ashton M. Getting rid of stupid stuff. N Engl J Med. 2018;379(19):1789–91. https://doi.org/10.1056/NEJMp1809698.
9. ECRI Institute. Top 10 patient safety concerns 2020. https://www.ecri.org/landing-top-10-patient-safety-concerns-2020
10. Bates D, Kuperman G, Wang S, et al. Ten commandments for effective clinical decision support: making the practice of evidence-based medicine a reality. J Am Med Inform Assoc. 2003;10(6):523–30. https://doi.org/10.1197/jamia.M1370.
11. Agency for Healthcare Research and Quality. Improving medication use and outcomes with clinical decision support: a step-by step-guide. https://digital.ahrq.gov/ahrq-funded-projects/current-health-it-priorities/clinical-decision-support-cds/chapter-1-approaching-clinical-decision/section-2-overview-cds-five-rights
12. Li RC, Wang JK, Sharp C, et al. When order sets do not align with clinician workflow: assessing practice patterns in the electronic health record. BMJ Qual Saf. 2019;28:987–96. https://doi.org/10.1136/BMJQS-2018-008968.

13. Kolwalcyzk L. Brockton hospital staff overlooked warning about a deadly allergy. 'Alert fatigue' may be to blame. Boston Globe. June 6, 2018. https://www.bostonglobe.com/metro/2018/06/06/brockton-hospital-staff-overlooked-warning-about-deadly-allergy-alert-fatigue-may-blame/TAecermEyROxRdcdMvyCvM/story.html
14. Lyell D, Magrabi F, Raban M, et al. Automation bias in electronic prescribing. BMC Med Inform Decis Mak. 2017;17:28. https://doi.org/10.1186/s12911-017-0425-5.

Patients and Families

9

Amy C. Drader

I spent the large majority of my life not thinking about healthcare, let alone interacting with the institution. Growing up, my parents, siblings, and I were very healthy. I could count on one hand the number of times I've been to a specialist. I married a man who had a similar background. When we had our first child, the pregnancy was typical and uneventful. We had a home birth. I remember this peaceful and calm experience initially laboring while watching the snowfall in our backyard. Certainly, when labor heated up, no one would have described me as calm. Yet, our son Harrison was born healthy and without event after 18 hours of labor with two midwives and my husband at my side.

Shortly after, I was hired at a pediatric hospital in learning and development. This was a thrilling opportunity being a new mom and now working with the world's best and brightest in pediatrics. I spent a career designing and delivering training on leadership and team development but in non-healthcare business settings or with the federal government. Those organizational structures and environments can be very similar. Healthcare was a whole other universe for me. So much so, I initially struggled with the ubiquitous terms people steeped in the industry take for granted,

A. C. Drader (✉)
Growth Partners Consulting,
Washington, DC, USA
e-mail: amy@growthpartnersconsulting.com

R. Roberts-Turner, R. K. Shah (eds.), *Pocket Guide to Quality Improvement in Healthcare*,
https://doi.org/10.1007/978-3-030-70780-4_9

like the difference between "inpatient" and "outpatient." I kept thinking to myself, "Aren't all patients in?" The meaning of those terms was not obvious to me. It took a solid 3 years for me to start to understand the experiences and challenges of this industry. My job was and still is to help healthcare employees work more effectively together.

When I became pregnant with our daughter Julia, everything changed.

At the 20-week ultrasound, Julia was diagnosed with myelomeningocele, or the most severe form of spina bifida. It was devastating. A neural tube defect, spina bifida occurs at the very initial stages when the baby's spine is formed. In Julia's case, her spine and nerves formed outside of her body as a result of an open lesion in her lower back. Julia also had hydrocephalus or a buildup of cerebral spinal fluid in her brain. We were terrified looking up information online and seeing the different ways our child's life could be impacted. We learned after another round of testing about fetal surgery. A procedure to close Julia's back while she was inside me – surgery on a human, inside a human. It seemed like science fiction. Our first birth, a home birth, involved the lowest level of technology possible. Our second birth went speeding to the opposite end of the spectrum.

When the nerves of the child's spine are exposed to amniotic fluid during pregnancy, additional damage is caused to the child's health. Fetal surgery closes the child's back in utero. By doing so, the damage is stopped. There are countless benefits to having the surgery. There are risks too.

This kind of operation puts two lives at stake. Over the course of 2 days, my own health was intensively evaluated and so was the baby's. In addition, my husband's health history was scrutinized and even our marriage. We were interviewed with a psychologist who was clearly seeking to understand if there were any signs of abuse or trauma that in some way could adversely impact the outcome of the surgery. The two-day evaluation process made it clear that this surgery was not something to consider lightly. When we learned of qualifying, we made the tough choice to move forward.

Experiencing something like fetal surgery is a level on its own. There is the terrifying and emotional stress of making that decision to have surgery, and that decision could result in losing the baby. It is rare but possible. A parent's mind will spiral, "What if I am responsible for losing our child?" As we weighed our decisions about the surgery, we met with countless people: maternal and fetal medicine specialists, neurosurgeons, genetic counselors, radiologists, neonatologists, nurses, psychologists, and socials workers. The hospital we were at was out of network. The insurance paperwork was incredible. We had inches thick file folders to keep track of everything. Feeling overwhelmed was an understatement.

Looking back, I was in 100% patient mode. I did not see myself also as a healthcare professional in the midst of fetal surgery, during recovery, birth, or even the first 6 months of Julia's life. During that time, we could barely keep up with the number of appointments we had. I was and still am grateful now to be working at the same institution where Julia receives care. The care we received for fetal surgery was fantastic, and the care we receive now is excellent as well. We have received quality care and have felt that we were the center of those care strategies.

Yet, this is not the experience of many parents. We belong to parent groups on social media, an excellent venue for sharing information and stories (though it has its pitfalls too) and have learned about a wide variety of approaches to care. **As patients and families, it is clear: the more involved we are, the more included we feel, and the better the care we receive.** Putting patients and families at the center of care is a core tenant of quality improvement. Yet, it had become abundantly clear through my many interactions as a parent and professional that patients and families do not intuitively know how to be involved, know the right questions to ask, or have the means to navigate the healthcare field. In addition, healthcare teams do not always have the knowledge and skills to effectively work together, let alone bring patients and families into the team as well.

The purpose of this chapter is to offer strategies to draw patients and families into the team-based approach to care, leveraging my experience as a parent of a medically complex child and as a team development professional. A framework for team-based care will first be introduced. Then, there will be brief discussion of just some of the obstacles that get in the way of teams working effectively together. The chapter concludes by elevating the framework to align with a list of questions to engage patients and families. The value of this framework is it can be used outside of patient care. Any team, regardless of industry, will benefit from this approach to working together.

When Julia was 16 months old she needed two surgeries. They were relatively minor but both required anesthesia and recovery time. We were nervous about both surgeries occurring within a short timeframe. During a conversation with her first surgeon, we mentioned Julia's need for the second surgery and described it to him. He then offered to team up with the other surgeon to perform both surgeries under the same sedation. It was a scheduling struggle at first. Finding operating room time and scheduling pre-op appointments while balancing surgeon availability with our own schedules was a challenge at best. Yet, we worked together to make it happen. Experiencing doctors and nurses working with us heightened the trust and confidence in our daughter's care.

"Team-based care" has been around for some time in medicine. Generally speaking, the goal of it is to best meet the needs of the patient as well as the family by making the patient a part of the team, not the object of the team.

I have learned through numerous conversations with healthcare providers that when people come together effectively as a team, those members are more engaged, overall satisfaction is improved, and those members want to remain on the team. They do not quit. Loyalty and commitment are fostered, and creativity is nurtured. Not only is team-based care an approach that provides better outcomes for patients and families but also for the team members.

To do this, it is important to know what working in an effective team looks like. There are fundamental principles that make teams high performing. I've spent a 20-year career in this field, and in some ways the basics are repeated over and over again in leadership and team development books. My intention here is not to recite the research in team development. Rather, there are basics that we all can list as being important to working together with others. These basic components are easily identified by just reflecting on our own experiences of working with others on a team.

Generally speaking, high-performing teams possess the following: clear goals, defined roles, conflict resolution, and feedback. The thread that ties it all together is communication: really good communication, not just reporting information back and forth but meaningful dialogue made up of asking questions and listening.

Here is a breakdown of what is involved in each component. This is not all inclusive. It is a general review of basic concepts.

Goals Everyone on the team knows what they are trying to achieve, in a specific way. The goals are aspirational and provide members a sense of connection to what they are working toward. As a parent I want to experience a group of people rally around the well-being of my child and my family. In order to rally, there has to be a goal. It describes or paints a picture of what is different as a result of working together.

Defined Roles Each member on the team is not only clear on their own role and what is expected but also the roles and expectations of each other. Assumptions fill the gaps if the team has not made these definitions obvious. Setting expectations early on with patients and families about their role and what it looks like is paramount in team-based care. Patients or parents will not naturally see themselves as having a part on the team at all. Discussing this and how the care team sees the patients contributing to the decisions will help draw them into the team in a more productive way.

Conflict Resolution No team has ever existed without conflict or disagreement. The teams that perform best are those that navigate it productively and talk about conflict before it comes up. They have a plan to resolve it before anyone disagrees. An important component of conflict resolution is empathy. Can the physician or nurse or technician step into the shoes of that parent and feel what they are feeling? It's emotional and, for some, uncomfortable ground. However, empathy shifts teams out of judgment and into understanding. When people understand each other, they work more effectively together, and they certainly resolve conflict faster.

Feedback Feedback is about improvement and most effective when it is expected and routine. Teams may dedicate certain time to discuss performance and use a format to do so such as Plus/Delta, a Lean methodology. The Plus side reveals what is going well. Delta or Δ refers to a symbol for change. This means the team discusses changes that can be made. These conversations are free of personality or gossip. These feedback conversations are centered on the care and are focused on improvement.

Communication This is the thread that ties it all together. Yet, it is probably the most difficult. Entire postdoctoral programs are dedicated to the study of communication, so clearly we will not discuss it all here. What I tend to advise the teams I work with and also try to model in my own interactions with Julia's providers are two basic communication tactics: ask questions and listen. When talking about goals, ask questions and listen. When defining roles, ask questions and listen. The crux of resolving conflict relies on asking questions and listening. The same goes for feedback. Clearly, at some point everyone on the team will need to state an opinion or make a decision. Do that. Then, pause, ask questions, and listen.

I would be remiss to not mention the role of a leader. It is well documented that leadership of the team is critical to its success. What gets tricky in healthcare is that team leadership and membership changes frequently. As a parent and employee, I quickly noticed how residents and fellows come and go. There are rotating shifts of nurses and other support staff, which often results in a different team in almost every appointment.

Generally speaking, the physician is almost always looked to as the leader of the team, regardless of reporting structure. This puts a greater expectation on the part of the physician to model the behaviors needed in the team. As a parent, I also look to the physician as the leader and hold an expectation for them to take that leadership role. But I also realized it's a tough spot to be in because of the lack of authority a physician has on overall team performance. In so many institutions, nurses report up to nursing, administration reports to administration, and physicians report up through other physicians. Yet, everyone is expected to work as a team despite many having different bosses and fighting institutionalized silos. The physician, who many look to as the leader, has very little authority over others.

This means everyone on the team is responsible for its success. This framework is designed to inform every person on the team what to do and how to do it. It is not dependent on a single leader. Teams certainly benefit from single leaders, but it's not always realistic or feasible in healthcare. So, healthcare teams all need to be equally informed on what actions to take for quality teamwork.

The purpose of this section is to describe team-based care and what the components of it look like: goals, defined roles, conflict resolution, and feedback with consistent communication threaded throughout the interactions. Team-based care yields better results, and we experienced that when Julia's surgeons teamed up for us to perform two surgeries under one sedation. However, it is not easy, and there are countless challenges and obstacles that hinder teams working together. The next section will address just that.

Julia regularly sees four to six different specialists. Thankfully, all six are in the same location, and the ideal is to see everyone in one visit every 6 months. All of her doctors and nurses recommend we group appointments into 1 day. This makes great sense and is ideal, especially for the parent. Yet, weekday clinics, appointment availability, more emergent cases, unexpected conflicts, sibling care, school activities, work schedules, available time off, and everyone's fortitude and attitude have to sync up to make it happen. It rarely does. For example, I spent at least 3 hours trying to schedule an ultrasound plus two clinic appointments for the same day. We got it done, and I received emailed confirmations for all three appointments. Yet, something happened with the ultrasound. We weren't on the schedule, and the rest of the timeslots were booked. It had something to do with one system not talking to another. I don't know. What I do know is that I had to waste 2 hours at the hospital with an 18 months old before the first clinic appointment. We also had to return the following week for the ultrasound.

There are countless obstacles in the way of creating a team-based care model. The example above is generally centered on scheduling and that is just one obstacle. Other challenges include complex health insurance, overwhelming medical information, paperwork and signatures needed – not to mention the constant stress and worry of being unwell or having an unwell or atypical child. Patients and families may very well be the most important members of the care team but also may be the ones most difficult to draw into that role.

The healthcare environment can be very intimidating, and as a parent, it is hard not to see yourself as anything other than an outsider. Even as a team development professional, I did not see myself as having a role on my daughter's care team. Both my husband and I were oblivious to it, especially when she was first born.

Very early in Julia's life, she was hospitalized. During rounds, the physicians and nurses would gather, stand in a circle, and talk without asking us any questions. They might smile and nod toward us, but that was it. We were literally outside their circle. We would eavesdrop but rarely understood the language and acronyms used. They were the experts, we were mere parents. In some ways, we conjured up this perception ourselves. If we had an urgent question, I believe we would have spoken up. But behaviors and posture, such as standing in a circle with backs and shoulders facing us, reinforced this impression of being excluded.

Certainly, there are instances where clinical providers may need to hold discussions without the patient or parent. We do not need to be involved in every discussion. Rather, if the parents are present, include them. Make a point to translate acronyms and complex medical terms into plain language to the parent. This might require identifying someone in rounds to take this role as well as carving out the time to do it.

Yet, this leads to another barrier, time. Never have we been more pressed for time in appointments than now. The pressure physicians and healthcare staff are under to create profitable clinics and drive productivity is significant. As an employee, I see it firsthand in meetings and financial report outs. What's today's census? Is it up? Is it down?

I have lunch with stressed colleagues who feel they are losing or have lost the joy of what brought them to medicine in the first place, the time and interaction with patients. A colleague of mine recently said, "I didn't become a doctor to spend my day arguing with insurance companies." Layer all the other stress on healthcare professionals – such as frustrations with the electronic health record, online reviews, administrative duties, regulatory and organizational change, scorecards, and reimbursements – and it's no wonder the patient and family interaction is decreased and in some instances even lost.

Patients and families feel it and see it. Brenda, a friend of mine who also has a child with spina bifida, talks about a physician they see who quadruple books her 8:00 AM appointments with less complex cases. Her strategy is to compensate for patients who are "no-show" as well as to move quickly through more cases in a short time. However, on the days everyone shows up to the 8:00 AM slot, it backs up the schedule. Clinic staffs mumble about it, and the frustration of other patients and families mounts throughout the day. The worst appointment to have is the 4:00 PM appointment. Everyone is tired, frustrated, abrupt, and running really, really late.

Brenda inevitably vents about the lack of time with the physician. She knows she only has 5 minutes before the doc is onto the next appointment, and often Brenda complains that if she just had another 5–10 minutes, she might have thought of the questions that came to her in the car ride home. I also believe that her physician, in many ways, feels the same. She would love to spend another 5–10 minutes with all of her patients. Doing so would reinforce who she truly is and why she became a pediatric physician in the first place.

Another major obstacle is racial, socioeconomic, and cultural disparities. My husband and I are white, well-educated, have insurance, and live in close proximity to the hospital. The large majority of our physicians and care providers look just like us. We have great privilege which makes getting the care we need for our daughter just plain easier. If a family is non-white, lives hours away, and has low income, inconsistent transportation, no insurance, limited education, multiple children to care for, jobs without leave, and/or language and cultural barriers, the obstacles to get any healthcare are great. Layer on a complex diagnosis, and it can feel impossible.

Team-based care is even more important to quality care given the very real disparities and biases that are at play. The fundamentals of communication in the framework (ask questions and listen) cannot be underestimated. An intensive care doctor I know well, Tamar, tells a story of witnessing biases at play in the care setting. Three residents were discussing a child who had not been visited by parents in 2 days. They were talking in pitying and judgmental tones regarding the lack of presence of a parent. Tamar, the attending and an exceptional teacher, approached them and asked, in a pleasant tone, "What do you know about this family?" They responded by speaking clinically of the child's diagnosis which wasn't her question. Tamar, who knew the family well, explained that the parent was single and working an hourly job and had very little leave time. In addition, she had two other school-age children to care for and support. The patient's siblings missed him terribly, and this mother was heartbroken to not be at the hospital with her child. "Yet, this mother entrusts us to care for her child and support her in every way we can."

As a parent, a logical next question is, what kind of care does a child receive if a parent is not at bedside? How are providers judging me, and how are decisions made if I can't be present with my child? Who's got my back? This is why a team-based approach is so important. Teams build relationships with each other and empathize. This model lends a structure and guide to providing the best possible care. Creating space to discuss the goals of working together, the roles everyone plays, and how to support each other, especially the parent.

The final challenge to be addressed is intended to call out the obvious: working in teams is hard, especially in healthcare. The dynamic nature of the environment with shifting staff, schedules, and patients along with ever-changing rules and regulations makes it a very complex environment. Hospital employees could find themselves working on a different team month to month, day to day, and even patient to patient. The members of the various teams could include a host of players – doctors, nurses, therapists, technicians, researchers, schedulers, specialists, social workers, and volunteers – and those players may have varying levels of training and education on how to actually work as a team. These are learned behaviors. Factor in varying personalities, egos, age groups, and stress, and it is no wonder we have teams that struggle.

Acknowledging the difficulty of working as a team is important. It means if we are on a team that is struggling, we are not alone. Each person bears a responsibility for making it successful, and the next section provides a framework to do just that.

Julia had a physical therapist that employed a team-based approach and set remarkable goals for her development. The therapist would ask us, "What do you want to see Julia doing in 6 months? Here are some options..." Many of those options I found unbelievable, such as independently crawling. Julia's head size was very large due to her hydrocephalus. She struggled to hold her head up to crawl, and her mobility from the waist down was so limited due to the L2 lesion on her back. I truly thought she would never crawl. The PT was optimistic and challenging. She not only pushed Julia but pushed us to think big for her. This meant we also pushed ourselves to maintain therapy at home, which supported and maybe at times accelerated her development. Julia became a speedy crawler by age two.

There is a wealth of research that describes what high-performing teams do. The question is how to engage patients and families knowing that if they are active members of the team, the care may very well be improved. From a parent's perspective, it is really quite simple: ask for our perspective, understand our circumstances, give us choices, and include us in the decisions. These needs are well in line with the framework offered in this chapter and support the tenants of patient-focused excellence. High-performing teams have clear goals, defined roles, conflict resolution, and feedback as well as strong communication (made up of asking questions and listening) woven throughout each component. Communication is that thread tying it all together.

In my work at the hospital, I regularly have staff coming to me with "Amy, I don't know what to say. Can you just give me the words?" In the spirit of this frequent request, the following table takes this concept to the next level by offering suggestions for how to engage the parent in the care team through conversation. Certainly, this is not an exclusive or even novel approach. The steps and language offered are common place. However, hearing these words, said this way, might influence parents to engage differently than they had before.

Weaving communication throughout each component of the framework, the following table lists each element and provides guidance entitled the "teaching moment." This creates context for the parent and provides an explanation for why these questions are asked. Being conscious of not sounding condescending is vital with teaching moments.

Then, after providing the instruction, there is a list of questions designed to draw the parent into the conversation. The point here is not to ask every single question. It is to provide a list of options to start a conversation and keep it going. Not all questions will be relevant or apply. Notice the questions are all open ended and the use of the pronouns "we" and "us." This is intentional to foster a team-based dialogue (Table 9.1).

This model can be applied outside of engaging with parents too. All teams benefit from leveraging this framework to take time to discuss how they work together. Ideally, if there is a leader of the team, that leader is the one to take the initiative to start these conversations. Yet, again, each member of the team plays a role in its success, so anyone can start these conversations. What is essential is for teams to intentionally set aside time to ask questions and listen to each other about each of the components of the framework. Generally speaking, the teams that openly discuss and plan their work using a framework like this will perform better than those who do not.

The purpose of this chapter is to offer strategies to draw parents into the team-based approach to care, leveraging my experience as a parent of a medically complex child and as a team development professional. The focus has been on quality care knowing that the more patients and families are involved, the more they are included, and better care is received.

Table 9.1 Engaging patients and families through conversation using the team development framework

Component	Conversation starters
Clear goals: The purpose of these questions is to inform the care team of what is important to the parent. Goals can then be defined leveraging everyone's input.	**Teaching moment:** When we're all on the same page with a common goal, we know we will create better care options for your child. We want to hear from you what goals you have for your child so that we can all work together to achieve them. Conversation starters: What do you want us to accomplish as a team? What does success look like? What is holding you back now? What has been hard to manage? What is going well? What about it makes it a success? What are you learning about your child's diagnosis? What have you researched or talked about with others? Who else supports you and your child's well-being? Tell me about your family.
Defined roles: The purpose of these questions is to understand what role the parent wants to or can play. It will also set the stage to inform the role the care team wants or needs the parent to play.	**Teaching moment:** You play a critical role on our team and we want to hear your perspective. We think it's important to understand each other's expectations and roles. We see you as a vital partner in the development of care plans. Conversation starters: What are your expectations for how we'll make decisions as a team? What role do you want to play in decision-making? Who are the other decision-makers involved in the care of your child? How do you want to include your child in the decisions? How would you like us to interact and communicate with your child versus communicating only with you? Who else is providing care, and what role do they play?

(continued)

Table 9.1 (continued)

Component	Conversation starters
Conflict resolution: The purpose of these questions is to discuss and address disagreement before it comes up.	**Teaching moment:** We will inevitably disagree and that's ok. That means we will make better decisions and identify better solutions for your child. If we talk about disagreeing before it comes up, we'll handle it together more effectively. When we disagree, we'll go back to our goals. Conversation starters: What experience do you have disagreeing with a nurse or a doctor? What is it like for you when you disagree? How should we handle disagreement? How do you prefer to share your opinions? In person or via email or text? What ideas do you have for us to handle disagreement effectively?
Feedback: The purpose of these questions is to invite feedback and set the context of improvement rather than criticism.	**Teaching moment:** Your opinion matters, and we want to hear how we're doing as a team. We will always be looking for ways to improve, and we'll routinely check in with you on progress. We also provide surveys, and we'd appreciate you sharing your feedback there as well. Conversation starters: What is going well with our work together? What can we improve? What should we start doing, stop doing, and continue doing? How well-informed do you feel about the care you're receiving? How would you evaluate our performance toward the goals we set? What aspects of our goals need to change in order to improve the care we provide?

The basic components of a successful team were presented: clear goals, defined roles, conflict resolution, and feedback with communication woven throughout each one. That communication is demonstrated by asking questions and listening. Certainly, there are plenty of obstacles that get in the way. The overwhelming nature of healthcare; an overall lack of time; racial, socioeconomic, and/or cultural disparities; or just the simple fact that working in teams is hard are all valid reasons to turn away from a team-based approach. Yet, as healthcare professionals we know that when the patients and families are engaged and involved, the outcomes are better.

Providers Are Key to Quality 10

Jessica A. Cronin and Srijaya K. Reddy

What Is QI? QI Is a Methodology to Improve the Care We Provide to Our Patients

As healthcare providers we work at the frontline – an operating room, hospital, or a clinic – and it is a hectic place. On any given day, the preoperative holding area is full of surgical patients who are waiting for surgery; patients wait in the emergency room needing to be triaged; clinics have a full schedule on top of squeezing in last-minute appointments for acutely ill patients. We have to be compliant with cumbersome documentation in electronic health records and complete other administrative tasks, which often takes time away from direct patient care [1]. Amidst the day-to-day grind, how do we make sure each patient receives the attention and care they deserve?

J. A. Cronin (✉)
Division of Anesthesiology, Pain, and Perioperative Medicine, Children's National Hospital, Washington, DC, USA
e-mail: jcronin@childrensnational.org

S. K. Reddy
Department of Anesthesiology, Division of Pediatric Anesthesiology, Monroe Carell Jr. Children's Hospital/Vanderbilt University Medical Center, Nashville, TN, USA
e-mail: srijaya.k.reddy@vumc.org

R. Roberts-Turner, R. K. Shah (eds.), *Pocket Guide to Quality Improvement in Healthcare*,
https://doi.org/10.1007/978-3-030-70780-4_10

First, we have to define what high-quality care is. The Institute of Medicine developed a framework to define high-quality healthcare, which has six aims: to be safe, effective, patient-centered, timely, efficient, and equitable [2]. We all entered the healthcare profession committed to providing this type of care to our patients. But unfortunately, this level of quality and consistency is not the experience for all patients [3]. Quality improvement (QI) is a tool that helps us to bridge the gap between what is happening and what patient care should be.

While we all learned anatomy, pharmacology, and physiology in our training, most of us we were not formally taught QI in school [4]. Developed by W. Edwards Deming and others, QI is the science of making changes that lead to improved patient health outcomes and enhanced delivery of patient care. This scientific process uses medical knowledge from empirical studies and implements change in a way that is effective in a specific, local care setting [5].

Quality improvement has several main components based on the IHI Model for Improvement [6]:

1. Set an aim – *What are we trying to accomplish?*
2. Select a measure – *How will we know that a change is an improvement? What measurement will show if you achieved your aim?*
3. Develop interventions – *What change can we make that will result in improvement of our measure?*
4. Implement interventions and follow up – *In a Plan-Do-Study-Act (PDSA) cycle, first plan, then implement an intervention, and then study if the intervention resulted in improvement and act based on that new information.*

QI Methodology Can Help You Achieve Specific Goals

You can apply this model in all sorts of settings, and it can even address problems outside of healthcare. We have used the PDSA cycle and this model for substantive QI projects; however for the sake of demonstrating the simplicity of this model, let us take potty training as a straightforward example. Years ago, we were preparing our son to go to preschool. While Jack was three and a half and otherwise ready to go to school, there was one requirement that he had not met yet – he had to be potty-trained. We had read all the books and tried all the gimmicks without much success. But with only 3 months until the start of preschool, we needed to confront potty training again with a fresh approach. Lucky for him (or maybe unlucky?), Jack had two parents who were anesthesiologists and also well versed in QI. Why not treat this problem like a QI project?

With this newly found structure, we got right to it. We had a clear aim (step 1): to have Jack potty-trained within 3 months. Jack was also on board because he was very excited to go to school like his older brother and understood that he needed to be potty-trained to start. Then, we defined our measure (step 2): the number of daily accidents. Our target was to reduce the number of daily accidents on average to less than one per day. Finally, we developed interventions (step 3) we thought might help us achieve our goals; we also asked Jack what he thought would help. Jack suggested that he should get a live dinosaur (which were extinct millions of years ago) each time he used the toilet instead of having an accident, but given the reality, we decided on dinosaur stickers instead. He would receive a dinosaur sticker if he said he had to go to the toilet and two stickers if he actually used the toilet. But after this sticker incentive intervention, Jack continued to have many daily accidents with no improvement. Rather than feeling personally defeated, we tried other interventions (promises of movies and stories, toys, timed visits to the toilet) and continued measuring daily accidents to evaluate how effective our interventions were (step 4). Eventually, we tried candy (M&Ms) as an incentive. Within 2 days, Jack's daily accident rate had cut in half, and soon enough accidents were so rare; Jack was ready for preschool! Now, I often use Jack's potty training experience to educate learners about QI. And, Jack still loves his candy, M&Ms.!

QI is more recognized to address specific problems in the clinical arena. For example, we were having an issue with hypothermia in our neonatal intensive care unit (NICU) patients undergoing surgery. As pediatric anesthesiologists we knew that hypothermia has been associated with increased mortality and higher rates of complications like sepsis, necrotizing enterocolitis, and bronchopulmonary dysplasia [7]. Despite this knowledge, 10% of these patients were returning to the NICU from the operating room (OR) hypothermic. We developed a multidisciplinary team of anesthesiologists, neonatologists, OR circulating nurses, surgical technicians, NICU nurses, and anesthesia technicians to help us solve this problem. Together, we defined the aim of this project to decrease the rate of hypothermia by half from 10% to 5%. We discussed reasons why we thought our smallest patients were getting cold in the OR, and then we identified interventions to address those causes, including (1) the development of a checklist to remind clinicians of all the tools that we have to keep infants warm as we had not previously been using all the tools at our disposal; (2) creating an improved process of temperature monitoring to ensure temperature was being measured appropriately and continuously from the time when the baby left the NICU until the time they returned to the NICU after surgery because we noted there were often periods when the patient's temperature was not being measured; and (3) increased transparency so all perioperative providers were aware of the current hypothermia rate and the goal rate for our NICU patients and to encourage awareness and engagement. We implemented these interventions and continued to measure the percentage of patients that were hypothermic (Fig. 10.1). The hypothermia rate decreased from 10% to 2% in 3 months! These interventions are still in place today as we strive to maintain a low rate of hypothermia in the postoperative period. Our anesthesiology division is now nationally recognized for excelling at temperature management for surgical NICU patients. QI was the framework to improve our NICU patient outcomes, and this same model has been applied at multiple institutions [8].

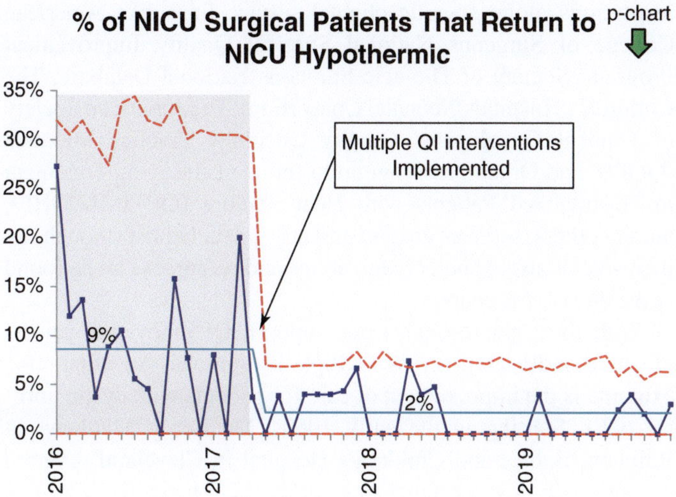

Fig. 10.1 Rate of hypothermic NICU surgical patients

QI Is Also Highly Effective When Used Across Multiple Institutions

The NICU temperature management example illustrates how clinicians can use QI to address specific outcomes in a relatively simple system involving a particular clinical setting over a relatively short time period. Processes get increasingly complicated when you consider more complex outcomes like population health, which can encompass healthcare provided across many years and involves multiple healthcare settings. The same methodology can be effective, but diverse collaboration and leadership are essential to develop and implement innovative ideas and effectively spread those interventions across multiple settings or institutions. There are a number of organizations that provide healthcare-related QI resources for the new QI learner as well as the expert, like the Institute for Healthcare Improvement. Successfully coordinated improvement processes across multiple institutions along specific clinical service lines like American College of Surgeons National Surgical Quality Improvement Program, Society of Thoracic Surgeons National Database, The Children's Hospitals Neonatal Consortium, The American Society of Clinical Oncologists' Quality Oncology Practice Initiative (QOPI), and Organized Program to Initiate Lifesaving Treatment in Hospitalized Patients with Heart Failure (OPTIMIZE-HF), among others, serve as great examples. A detailed list (though not inclusive of all) of such organizations and resources can be found at the end of this chapter.

With the right resources and support, QI innovation can be effective and extend across multiple institutions. An often-cited example is the improvement of care for patients with cystic fibrosis (CF). Starting in the early 1960s, Dr. Leroy Matthews at Rainbow Babies and Children's Hospital in Cleveland reported exceptionally low mortality rates in their CF patients. With data collected by the Cystic Fibrosis Foundation, physicians learned that while most patients had a median life span of 12 years in 1964, Dr. Matthews' patients were consistently living to the age of 21 years [9]. Dr. Matthews' unique treatment plan, including prophylactic interventions for his patients before they were even symptomatic, became the gold standard for how to care for patients with CF. Using the same database about mortality and quality of life metrics, institutions continue to implement advancements to how they cared for CF patients today [10]. So while individual QI projects may start out as projects focused on a narrow aim like decreasing hypothermia in NICU surgical patients at one institution, they can provide structure for improving outcomes for a whole population.

Clinicians Are Uniquely Positioned to Engage in QI

Physicians like Dr. Matthews, you, and I are on the frontline. While we have the evidence-based knowledge of what consistent, excellent care for our patients should be, we also recognize how challenging it is to provide it because we can identify obstacles every day. We are aware of the distinct steps that need to be done correctly to complete tasks effectively and reliably – from safely placing a central line or administering the appropriate antibiotic to a septic patient in a timely fashion to managing glucose levels in diabetic inpatients or maximizing the number of pediatric outpatients who are up-to-date on their vaccinations. We can use this in-the-weeds knowledge to identify QI interventions that would make it easier for us, as providers, and the entire healthcare system to do the right thing every time.

QI Interventions Can Be Low-Tech

QI interventions can take on very different forms depending on the clinical need and ingenuity of the QI team. For example, consider the intensive care unit (ICU) environment. Every day, there is a long list of complicated tasks to complete for multiple critically ill patients. It is easy to get distracted amidst several priorities that are both concurrent and urgent. QI can help in this scenario, and the interventions don't need to be highly technical. Dr. Peter Pronovost, an anesthesiologist and critical care physician at Johns Hopkins Hospital, was frustrated about the high rate of central line-associated blood infections. Central line catheter infections are associated with severe complications like sepsis and death, as well as increased costs (about $45,000 per infection), and studies show that the majority of infections that happen are absolutely preventable. Dr. Pronovost borrowed wisdom from the aviation industry and developed a checklist: (1) wash your hands, (2) use full-barrier precautions, (3) prepare insertion site with chlorhexidine antiseptic, (4) avoid femoral site for insertion, and (5) remove unnecessary lines. Prior to implementation of Dr. Pronovost's checklist, one of these steps was skipped almost 40% of the time each time a central line was placed, even though ICU clinicians knew that these steps were effective and were not intentionally trying to provide suboptimal care! After multiple interventions were implemented, including the checklist, the rate of infections from central lines dropped 60% [11]. It is important to emphasize that the checklist was not implemented unaided; other interventions were necessary to support high-quality care associated with central line placement [12]. Nonetheless, Dr. Pronovost showed us that as frontline workers and clinical leaders, we can identify barriers to providing optimal care and work as part of a team to overcome those barriers.

QI Interventions Can Be Higher-Tech Too

Solutions to suboptimal care can be technological developments as well. In the 1950s, the field of anesthesiology had a problem – patients were dying, and dying often. In the 1950s and 1960s, anesthesia caused death in approximately 6 out of every 10,000 anesthetics and was often due to equipment misuse. That risk of death from anesthesia was 50 times worse than skydiving [13]! Thankfully, safety in anesthetic care over the subsequent 50 years improved tremendously. There has been a 10- to 20-fold decrease in morbidity and mortality from anesthesia-related causes [14]. While multiple innovations were responsible for the decreased in anesthesia-related risk, technological advancements in the design and function of the anesthesia, including the invention of the oxygen fail-safe device, are ultimately what made anesthesia safer for patients. Anesthesiologists use this machine not only to ventilate anesthetized patients but also to deliver gases to maintain patients under general anesthesia. In the 1950s, it could also easily deliver a hypoxic gas mixture to the patient if the anesthesiologist selected the incorrect setting for the gas. For example, nothing prevented the machine from accidently delivering 100% nitrous oxide (0% oxygen) to an anesthetized patient other than a vigilant anesthesiologist. Furthermore, diagnosis of hypoxia was often delayed in the absence of modern monitoring equipment. The American Society of Anesthesiologists did not require electrocardiogram for intraoperative monitoring until the 1970s. Pulse oximetry was adopted in the 1990s, and CO_2 capnography was not universally utilized until the early 2000s.

In fact, this exact scenario of accidental hypoxic gas delivery occurred repeatedly. After two patients died from hypoxia and a third experienced permanent brain damage due to inadvertent delivery of hypoxic gas mixtures at Columbia University in New York City, an anesthesiologist, Dr. Robert Epstein, and Arnold Lee, an engineer, developed a fail-safe device within the anesthesia machine. It ensured that a minimum of amount of oxygen must be delivered at all times and was eventually mandated by regulatory bodies and required for all anesthesia machines [15]. The fail-safe component was the first of many changes made to the anesthesia machine to improve patient safety; this innovation made it easier to do the right thing – to always deliver a gas mixture with sufficient oxygen when ventilating a patient.

Problems that once seemed impossible to fix, like preventable central line infections and high mortality due to anesthesia, can be addressed with small, incremental steps and iterative PDSA cycles within the IHI Model for Improvement. Further, from potty training to technological upgrades in anesthesia machines, QI can incorporate all sorts of interventions. People on the frontline like Dr. Epstein with the fail-safe device and Dr. Matthews with CF care not only defined problems in their practice and identified interventions but also implemented successful solutions that improved outcomes. They serve as an inspiration for us as we face today's challenges.

QI Is a Team Sport

As the stories in this chapter show, QI can lead to dramatic improvements in the care we provide our patients. But healthcare leaders like Drs. Epstein, Pronovost, and Matthews did not work alone. They were a part of a care team, working alongside nurses, other physicians, technicians, respiratory therapists, and many others who work together to take care of patients. As medical students most of us were not formally taught how to be effective clinical care team leaders. Instead, we often learned on the fly through our training. Some of my greatest teachers were experienced nurses I worked with as an intern. They taught me how the process of patient care actually worked in the hospital as I stumbled through my first admissions for heart failure, pneumonia, and acute kidney failure. Each clinical team member offers a unique expertise and perspective as we work together to care for patients with complex needs.

QI is also a team sport. As you consider your aim – your goal of what are you trying to accomplish – consider the system of people that relates to that aim. Who will be affected by the change? Engagement of those involved in all parts of the process – such as nurses, social workers, technicians, or administrative staff – is not suggested but required to make change possible and sustainable. Further, QI teams must contain diverse expertise in QI, clinical care, as well as leadership within the organization.

Emotional Intelligence Is Crucial for Successful QI

Together with your team, you will identify obstacles to achieving your aim and interventions that will help you overcome them. Differences in opinion within your team are good! The process of integrating these different perspectives will lead the team to consider all types of solutions that may not have otherwise have been considered.

Even when your QI team agrees on appropriate interventions, implementing QI is hard because it often involves a change in behavior. Chip and Dan Heath, in their book *Switch*, argue that emotions can overwhelm any rational thought when it comes to how people behave. In their model, there are two parts to every person. There is the emotional, gut-response side (the Elephant) and the rational, logical side (the Rider of the Elephant). Most of us think that the Rider controls the Elephant, but ultimately it is the other way around. A perfect example is going on a diet. The Rider wants better health, while the Elephant loves cookies – I don't have to tell you which side eventually wins! To successfully lose weight or improve health, you have to align the Elephant with the Rider [16].

We, clinicians, are comfortable talking to the Rider. We reference scientific articles, data, or information to justify what we do, but that is often not enough to implement permanent behavior changes in ourselves or our colleagues. We forget to engage the

Elephant. For example, prior to start of my QI project to reduce hypothermia in NICU surgical patients at our institution, our anesthesiologists were already aware of the evidence that showed the association between hypothermia with morbidity and mortality. Yet, we still had a high rate of hypothermia in our patients. Part of the QI project was to transition an aspect of our identity as anesthesiologists from providers who get patients through surgery to clinicians that continue to provide many different aspects of medical management for NICU surgical patients continuously throughout the perioperative period, including temperature management.

So how do we engage both sides – the Rider and the Elephant – to achieve QI? One way is to make the interventions into small, easy steps. Dr. Pronovost did this with his checklist for central line placement. He showed that following five easy steps decreases the rate of central line infections. Another approach is to change the environment to make it much easier to do the right thing. Dr. Epstein did this when he created an anesthesia safety device that makes it much more difficult to deliver hypoxic gas mixtures to patients. You can also be more effective when you have a clear plan with concrete steps. Going back to the diet example, just saying you want to lose weight without any clear next steps is not enough. You can be more effective when you have specific, reachable goals in terms of what and how much to eat as well as exercise targets. Dr. Matthews did the same in CF care when he showed that particular pulmonary treatments like chest physiotherapy, aerosolized treatments, and humidified air improved survival when given prophylactically as soon as a diagnosis was made as opposed to when only given to treat obstructive or infectious pulmonary symptoms. Dr. Matthews gave the rest of the medical community a clear path to better outcomes for CF patients, and within 6 years, the predicted age of survival increased by 4 years nationally – a dramatic change in a short amount of time! All these examples illustrate that there are various strategies available to achieve permanent behavior change for QI. Flexibility is essential as you think about which approach may be best based on the key stakeholders involved and the interventions you wish to implement.

There Will Be Stumbles Along the Way, But That Is Part of QI

We physicians hate to fail. Through our training, we have been tremendously focused on success. We got into medical school. We achieved high scores on countless tests. We completed a grueling residency and perhaps additional training. But there were failures along the way too that we often don't reflect on. Likewise, when I watched my then 12-month-old Jack learning to walk, he fell countless times, but every time, he would get back up and try again. Jack didn't look at each fall as a sign that he would never be able to walk. While as a parent, I could have done without some of the bigger bruises and emotional meltdowns that came with certain falls, I saw how Jack used the experience of each fall to try again more effectively. We encourage you to think about QI the same way. Failure is a necessary, expected part of each QI project just like falling is part of learning to walk. Use each stumble in your QI work to figure out how to do it better with each attempt.

QI Is an Effective Tool for Meaningful, Permanent Change: This Book Will Help You Do It!

This book gives you the tools to ensure patients get the high-quality care they deserve. Just like medicine, QI is a tool that mixes standardization of approach with need for creativity for solutions. It is often said that medicine is a combination of art and science – QI is the art and science of change.

References

1. Joukes E, et al. Time spent on dedicated patient care and documentation tasks before and after the introduction of a structured and standardized electronic health record. Appl Clin Inform. 2018;9(1):46–53.
2. Committee on Quality Health Care in America, Institute of Medicine. Crossing The Quality Chasm: a New Health System for the 21st Century. Washington, D.C.: National Academy Press, 2001.

3. McGlynn EA, et al. The quality of health care delivered to adults in the United States. N Engl J Med. 2003;348(26):2635–45.
4. Headrick LA, et al. Results of an effort to integrate quality and safety into medical and nursing school curricula and foster joint learning. Health Aff (Millwood). 2012;31(12):2669–80.
5. Batalden PB, Davidoff F. What is "quality improvement" and how can it transform healthcare? Qual Saf Health Care. 2007;16(1):2–3.
6. Institute for Healthcare Improvement. How to improve. http://www.ihi.org/resources/Pages/HowtoImprove/default.aspx. Accessed 1 July 2020.
7. Lyu Y, et al. Association between admission temperature and mortality and major morbidity in preterm infants born at fewer than 33 weeks' gestation. JAMA Pediatr. 2015;169(4):e150277.
8. Brozanski BS, et al. STEPP IN: working together to keep infants warm in the perioperative period. Pediatrics. 2020;145(4):e20191121.
9. Warwick WJ. Cystic fibrosis: nature and prognosis. Minn Med. 1967;50(7):1049–53.
10. Gawande A. Better: a surgeon's notes on performance. 1st ed. New York: Metropolitan; 2007. x, 273 p.
11. Berenholtz SM, et al. Eliminating catheter-related bloodstream infections in the intensive care unit. Crit Care Med. 2004;32(10):2014–20.
12. Bosk CL, et al. Reality check for checklists. Lancet. 2009;374(9688): 444–5.
13. United States Parachute Association. https://uspa.org/Find/FAQs/Safety. Accessed 22 May 2020.
14. Cooper JB, Gaba D. No myth: anesthesia is a model for addressing patient safety. Anesthesiology. 2002;97(6):1335–7.
15. Epstein RM, et al. Prevention of accidental breathing of anoxic gas mixtures during anesthesia. Anesthesiology. 1962;23:1–4.
16. Heath C, Heath D. Switch: how to change things when change is hard. 1st ed. New York: Broadway Books; 2010. 305 p.

Selected Recommended Reading About Quality Improvement

Bisognano MA, Kenney C. Pursuing the triple aim seven innovators show the way to better care, better health, and lower costs. San Francisco: Jossey-Bass; 2012.

Deming WE. The new economics for industry, government, education. Cambridge, MA: Massachusetts Institute of Technology, Center for Advanced Engineering Study; 1993. xii, 240 p.

Heath C, Heath D. Made to stick: why some ideas survive and others die. 2008 Random House hardcover ed. New York: Random House; 2008. 323 p.

Heath C, Heath D. Switch: how to change things when change is hard. 1st ed. New York: Broadway Books; 2010. 305 p.

Kenney C. Transforming health care: Virginia Mason Medical Center's pursuit of the perfect patient experience. Boca Raton: CRC Press; 2011. xxii, 223 p.

Kohn LT, Corrigan J, Donaldson MS. To err is human: building a safer health system. Washington, DC: National Academy Press; 2000. xxi, 287 p.

Langley GJ. The improvement guide: a practical approach to enhancing organizational performance. 2nd ed. San Francisco: Jossey-Bass; 2009. xxi, 490 p.

Nelson EC, Batalden PB, Godfrey MM. Quality by design: a clinical microsystems approach. 1st ed. Lebanon/San Francisco: Center for the Evaluative Clinical Sciences at Dartmouth; Jossey-Bass/Wiley; 2007. xliv, 459 p.

Provost LP, Murray SK. The health care data guide: learning from data for improvement. 1st ed. San Francisco: Jossey-Bass; 2011. xxviii, 445 p.

Selected Organizations That Focus on Quality Improvement

Agency for Healthcare Research and Quality. https://www.ahrq.gov/
Institute for Healthcare Improvement. http://www.ihi.org
National Association for Healthcare Quality. https://nahq.org/
National Quality Forum. https://www.qualityforum.org
The Deming Institute. https://deming.org/
The Joint Commission. https://www.jointcommission.org
The Leapfrog Group. https://www.leapfroggroup.org/

Nurses Protect Patients 11

Reneè Roberts-Turner
and Ana Figueroa-Altmann

Florence Nightingale pioneered the quality improvement journey in nursing. In 1859, Nightingale cared for soldiers injured during the Crimean War and quickly recognized that they were dying from illnesses, not their initial war injuries. Diseases such as cholera, typhoid, and other infectious illnesses killed scores of soldiers. Today, these illnesses would be recognized as hospital-acquired infections. Nightingale recognized that these deaths were linked to lack of hand hygiene, poor ventilation, lack of bathing the patients, dirty linens, as well as a decrease in air exchanges within the environment due to a lack of space between patients. The first quality improvement ideas in nursing focused on maintaining a cleaner patient care environment; procedures implemented by Nightingale included: standardization of linen changes, use of clean water, surgical instrument cleaning processes, standardization of bathing patients, and handwashing. Nightingale's improvement efforts reduced the mortality rate

R. Roberts-Turner (✉)
Division of Nursing, Children's National Health System,
Washington, DC, USA
e-mail: rrturner@childrensnational.org

A. Figueroa-Altmann
Department Patient Safety Officer, Children's Hospital of Philadelphia,
Philadelphia, PA, USA
e-mail: altmann@email.chop.edu

R. Roberts-Turner, R. K. Shah (eds.), *Pocket Guide to Quality Improvement in Healthcare*,
https://doi.org/10.1007/978-3-030-70780-4_11

from 60% to 42% to 2% [1, 2]! Quality improvement efforts remain imperative today within the nursing practice as our goal continues to be to keep our patients safe. The nursing process is the model that every nurse is trained to use to provide care. We have found that the link between the nursing process and the Model for Improvement is a unique and simple way to teach and apply quality improvement within the discipline of nursing.

The steps in the Model for Improvement align with the steps of the nursing process. The nursing process is a systematic standard core model that every nurse is trained to use to provide care to patients. The nursing process involves collecting and analyzing information, with the ultimate goal being to deliver patient-focused, holistic care. This five-step process includes assessment, nursing diagnosis, planning, implementation, and evaluation. The nursing process is the foundation for how nurses provide reasoned care to our patients and is the backbone of our clinical decision-making. Each step in the five-step nursing process builds upon the previous step. The nursing process is also the foundation for nursing care delivery as it allows nurses to individualize, contextualize, and prioritize problem areas that require intervention for improving the outcomes of nursing care.

The Model for Improvement, which will be referenced moving forward as the quality improvement (QI) process, can also be described using five action steps that align with the nursing process conceptually. At the point of care, the QI process has been shown to be effective in making sustainable improvements in a short period. The natural connection of the QI process to the nursing process speaks to the usability of the QI process, as a framework for nurses to use to improve care delivery [3] (Table 11.1).

Nurses must consistently seek to make improvements in the healthcare environment to ensure the best clinical outcomes for patients and families. The process of continuous improvement in nursing can be achieved by routinely evaluating the patient care delivery system, with a goal to ensure staff, patients, and their families are safe and obtain the expected outcomes [4]. Using the QI process is one way to examine our structures and processes in our pursuit of positive outcomes for patients, families, and staff. Understanding how each care team member's practices impact patients' care outcomes is the first essential step to consistently providing the best and most reliable patient care available.

Table 11.1 The steps of the nursing process and the phases of the quality improvement process

Process steps and actions	
Nursing	Quality improvement (QI)
Assessment Collecting and documenting data about the patient.	**Analyze** Examining the available data to determine and confirm that a problem exists and also to identify the scope of the problem
Nursing diagnosis Using the patients' needs and responses to queries to establish a nursing diagnosis	**Define and develop the problem** Identifying the scope and specifying metrics to make the problem measurable and providing an explanation as to what is needed to make actual improvements
Planning Identifying goals for the patient to establish a focused plan of care	**Design interventions** Identifying interventions and selecting those which are achievable and have the highest impact; design the procedures to be implemented
Implementation Completing nursing actions to implement the plan of care	**Implement** Implementing the above interventions
Evaluation Identify whether or not the preset care goals have been achieved by monitoring both the delivered care and the outcomes of the care	**Measure, spread, and sustain** Measuring the outcomes of the interventions

The next part of this chapter will define and describe the five action steps of the nursing process and the QI process. Examples for each action step will be provided to demonstrate the nurses' role in the QI process as a systematic approach to improve patient outcomes.

Assessment/Analyze

A comprehensive nursing assessment involves the collection of information, which is provided by the patient and/or the family, other healthcare providers, and medical records and observed by the nurse. This discovery phase of the nursing process involves the collection of data to include subjective patient-reported information and objective, observable data. The assessment is most successful when there is clear communication between the nurse and the patient and or family. The data collection includes psychological, economic, spiritual, and lifestyle factors. The second component of the nursing assessment involves the analysis and interpretation of the collected data, which allows the information to be presented in a meaningful way.

Like the nursing process, the nurse's role in the QI process involves analyzing data to identify a problem related to care delivery, the work environment, or patient experience. This can be accomplished by recognizing mistakes and identifying when there are too many steps in the process or when a process is too complicated. Below is an example of clinical nurses using data to identify interventions related to nursing care.

Example Nursing Analyze

Clinical nurses were involved in the evaluation of patient safety data in one of the intensive care units with regard to eliminating harm to patients from unintended extubations (UE), a nationwide patient safety issue that extends length of stay and increases healthcare costs due to the dislodgement of an endotracheal tube (ETT) before the decision is made by the medical team to remove the tube. The clinical nurses recognized this as an important safety issue on the unit and reviewed monthly UE data and recognized an increase in the NICU rate of UEs per 100 ventilator days to 1.11.

The focus of QI can involve fixing a current or designing a new system or process. Whether attempting to fix or design your system or process, the questions asked to identify the problem often differ. When looking to fix a current system or process, answering the following questions can help identify the problem:

- What worries you?
- What makes you believe there is an easier way to get the expected outcomes?
- Are we "working hard and not smart"?
  Are we failing to meet practice standards? [5, 6].

The step of identifying and defining the problem is crucial to the improvement work. Once the specific problem is detected, the focus of the project may be directed toward implementing the needed change or putting in place a new design for the system or process.

Nursing Diagnosis/Define and Develop the Problem

The nursing diagnosis provides overall direction, is the foundation for the nurses' care plan, and determines the course of treatment. The nursing diagnosis outlines the actual problem as well as any potential problems that the patient may be at risk for developing. The nursing diagnosis is a statement that includes the assessment of the problem and needs of the patient. Like the nursing process, the nurse's role in the QI process involves the nurse identifying, specifying, and then communicating the problem. Defining the problem explains what is needed to make actual improvements.

A problem statement must be a succinct, clear, nonjudgmental statement of the problem. A strong problem statement will allow you to focus the work and guide the improvement process. Once the problem statement has been identified, the understanding of the problem needs to be refined and the scope of the problem defined. Examples of problem statements which are not succinct, precise, or nonjudgmental include the following:

- The nurses feel like there isn't enough staff.
- The unit clerks are rude.
- You can never get help from the lean department.
- "We never see our leader, she's just not interested in us, she is always in her office with the door closed."

With the problem well identified, you will next develop an aim.

The aim statement is an explicit statement summarizing what a team hopes to achieve. It guides your work by providing a vision of what success looks like. The aim statement is time-specific and concise while identifying the affected population. It should include data and numeric goals that can be reliably measured. This information helps determine if implementing a change is an actual improvement [5, 6].

In summary, the aim statement must include the following:

- What the project will increase or decrease
- Group or population the project will affect
- Baseline (from what) and goal (to what)
- Timeframe written as a date (accomplish by when and sustain for how long) [6]

Example Nursing Define and Develop the Problem

Nurses on the nursing skin team recognized an upward trend in noninvasive respiratory device-related pressure injuries. Over the prior three prevalence studies, unique patient data revealed 75% of all respiratory device-related pressure injuries were attributed to noninvasive respiratory devices. These specific pressure injuries also accounted for one-quarter of hospital-acquired pressure injuries (HAPIs).

Problem statement: 75% of all respiratory device-related pressure injuries were attributed to noninvasive respiratory devices.

Aim statement: Decrease the rate of noninvasive respiratory device-related pressure injuries for all inpatients from 67% to 0% by December 2019 and sustain for 6 months.

Planning/Design Interventions

The development of a care plan is the next step of the nursing process after the nursing diagnosis has been established. Creating a care plan involves using information from the nursing assessment and diagnosis, identifying measurable outcomes, and planning nursing interventions. This plan is created with the patient and it is prioritized by addressing life-threating needs first. Evidence is used to establish interventions; measurable short- and long-range goals are established for each problem. The plan takes into consideration the patient's discharge needs, as well as ensuring the patient will be able to function, to the best of their ability, at the time of discharge.

Mirroring the nursing process, the nurse is an active team member in the design of interventions. Plan-Do-Study-Act (PDSA) is a method used to rapidly determine if an implemented change is working and allows you to take action, if it is not. Change is tested on a small scale. The change is then refined and tested again, until viable solutions are identified, and it is ready for broader implementation. The goal is to bring knowledge into action, versus discovering a single change that works best. The small test of change includes four steps:

1. Plan: By planning the intervention
2. Do: Trying the intervention
3. Study: Observing the results
4. Act: Acting on the learnings

In the nursing process, the nurse is responsible for identifying and beginning to plan for the discharge needs of a patient. Thoughtful and early discharge planning increases the likelihood that patients will be successful with their care needs after discharge. Using the same frame of thought early in the QI process, the nurse and QI team should be sure to identify strategies that will result in the sustainability of interventions. The intentional early focus on sustaining change ensures that the outcomes associated with the changes are maintained. Too often, interventions are put in place that are not sustainable because of the following:

- Various structures (reporting structures, how the unit is configured)
- Processes (how information is documented, the steps or processes followed by another department)
- Culture (what staff feel is important, how they work together)

Example Nursing Design Interventions

Two specialty clinics have an interprofessional team delivering a variety of services and care in a fast-paced and busy ambulatory setting. The complexity of these clinic structures and services frequently results in appointment delays for patients and their families. Nurses in these clinics witness incidences of patient and family dissatisfaction related to delays and shared these concerns with the educator and their nursing leadership. In addition the Press Ganey scores indicated a need to improve the Press Ganey "Information about Delays" question.

Nurses from two different specialty clinics and a nurse practitioner worked closely with one of their educators regarding their concerns in an effort to pinpoint the real delays within the two clinics based on recent patient satisfaction scores. Nurses identified ineffective closed-loop communication within the interprofessional team as a major factor in not properly informing patients and families regarding delays in appointments. The educator shared a literature review with the group of clinical nurses which revealed numerous findings suggesting that closed-loop communication could serve as an evidence-based change for the nurses to implement within their respective interprofessional teams and with patients and their families.

The nurses gathered feedback from stakeholders (staff, patients, and families) about their view of what influenced patient and family dissatisfaction in the ambulatory setting. This feedback revealed inadequate communication among clinical staff, resulting in decreased or disjointed communication to patients and families. The clinical nurses developed a system to communicate clinic flow to patients, families, and clinic staff using a standardized whiteboard and a traffic light system in their two clinics.

Implementation/Implement

The implementation of the care plan allows for continuity of care. The plan ensures that patient care is implemented according to the care plan during the hospitalization and in preparation for discharge. Care is documented in the patient's record. Interventions and responses to the interventions are carefully documented. The outcomes of care are evaluated, and new plans are created as needed. In the QI process, interventions are implemented locally. This step involves anchoring the new approach into the culture of the unit/ department. Implementation in the QI process requires the execution and collection of data associated with the change in one unit/department.

Example Nursing Design Interventions

The intravenous (IV) team nurses were experiencing a high demand for phlebotomy laboratory draws needed during the hours of approximately 6:00 pm to 6:00 am which was potentially inhibiting the IV team's primary responsibility to patient care and IV therapy. This identified an operational gap in phlebotomy services which could potentially delay decision-making, timely treatment, and/or patient discharge when adequate resources were not available to meet this operational need.

Nursing leadership requested the IV Team nurses track each time they performed phlebotomy and the related details which revealed that the IV team nurses performed a total of 103 phlebotomy lab draws in one week, in addition to their assigned care. Of the 103 phlebotomy lab draws, 65% were drawn, while phlebotomy services were scheduled. The nurse leader and clinical nurses collaborated and evaluated the data with the lab leadership team. The team examined the current practice and created and implemented improved processes for identifying the accurate flow for phlebotomy and increased staff awareness of stat (immediate) lab draw times. The new process ensured better alignment of operations and patient needs. The team was able to reduce the average number of requests directed to the IV team from 20 to 4 per day, which demonstrated an 80% improvement and reduced inefficiencies for the IV team nurses during open phlebotomy hours.

Evaluation/Measure, Spread, and Sustain

The effectiveness of nursing interventions is monitored continuously. This allows for opportunities for modifications of the care plan as needed. The patients' verbal and nonverbal responses observed by the nurse and other caregivers inform how effective the nursing interventions have been and can be used to formulate necessary modifications to the plans.

Spread, measure systemically, and sustain is the final step of the QI process and involves standardizing interventions to spread to applicable areas within the organization. This step helps with the enculturation and standardization of processes. Spreading involves anchoring the new approach into the culture by implementing the new process in applicable areas. Implementation and communication should occur thoughtfully and deliberately, until implemented organization-wide.

Once interventions have been implemented, continuous monitoring of performance is necessary to ensure the desired changes are being achieved. This requires monitoring the data on a pre-established frequency [7]. Clinical nurses provide direct patient care, and as part of this role, clinical nurses are aware of and assess effectiveness of nursing practice. This role function equips clinical nurses with the knowledge and expertise needed to identify ways to support continuous monitoring of performance.

Example Nursing Measure, Spread, and Sustain

Clinical nurses are empowered to advocate, not only for their patients but also for themselves. Clinical nurses' advocacy supports a culture of safety. Supporting a culture of safety can support efforts to address the needs of the growing behavioral health population and the increased risk potential toward nurses in the workplace.

During a staff meeting, nurses in the emergency department (ED) shared their anecdotal conclusion that the incident of assaults resulting in injury to nurses was high. The nurse manager shared that she and the leadership team would look at the incident reports and bring that actual rate of assaults resulting in injury to nurses to the next staff meeting. At the meeting, the manager shared that the actual rate of assaults resulting in injury to nurses for the ED was 5.14 per 100 incident reports for the last month. One nurse shared that in her previous organization, they used Kevlar sleeves to improve workplace safety for nurses and frontline staff. Kevlar sleeves are personal protective equipment (PPE) that add a layer of protection and play a large role in preventing bites and scratches in nursing personnel. The ED clinical nurses, nurse educators, and leaders conducted product trials through involvement in the organization's products committee and chose the preferred product. Education was provided to nursing representatives from the ED.

After a month of use in the ED, the incident rate of assaults resulting in injury to nurses decreased to 1.05 per 100 incident reports. The ED educators presented the early outcomes associated with Kevlar sleeves' use at the organizational nurse educator meeting. The decision was made that Kevlar sleeves would be used in all inpatient and outpatient areas that routinely care for patients with behavioral health diagnoses. Education was provided to nursing representatives from the unit educators. After spreading Kevlar sleeves usage to all applicable units, the incidence of the rate of assaults resulting in injury to nurses for the ED had been eliminated. The organizational data was trended monthly by the educators and decreased from 2.14 per 100 incident reports to 0.50 per 100 incidents (see graph 1 trended data).

Nurses are responsible for nursing outcomes of care while creating a positive, collaborative relationship with the patient as well as the patient's family. To do this, nurses must consistently seek to make improvements in the healthcare environment to ensure the best outcomes for patients and families. The steps in the nursing process align with the steps of the QI process, making the QI process a useful tool for the discipline of nursing to learn, embrace, and utilize on a daily basis.

References

1. Gill CJ, Gill GC. Nightingale in Scutari: her legacy reexamined. Clin Infect Dis. 2005;40(12).
2. Karimi H, Masoudi AN. Florence Nightingale: the mother of nursing. Nurse Midwifery Stud. 2015;4(2) https://doi.org/10.17795/nmsjournal29475.
3. Barker B. Quality improvement and the nursing process: what's the relationship? Ohio Nurs Rev. 2017;92(4).
4. Weiner BJ. A theory of organizational readiness for change. Implement Sci. 2009;4(67).
5. Connelly LM. Overview of Quality Improvement. Medsurg Nurs. 2018;27(2).
6. Institute for Healthcare Improvement. Science of Improvement: Setting Aims. http://www.ihi.org/resources/Pages/HowtoImprove/ScienceofImprovementSettingAims.aspx
7. Donabedian A. An introduction to quality assurance in healthcare. New York: Oxford Press; 2003.

12 Middle Management: Where the Rubber Meets the Road

Tina Kunze Humbel and Sharon Bostic

Quality improvement processes can serve as a powerful tool to foster engagement, establish goals, and serve as a catalyst for a department to establish an identity and to shape the culture of the work environment. In this chapter, we will discuss a handful of vital tools to begin the task of fostering the basic tenets used in quality improvement to foster your role as the middle manager. These tenets are a guideline to individualize an effective approach for you to use with both your direct reports and upper leaders.

Effective Communication

The middle manager's role in facilitating change at the department level starts with effectively translating the organization's goals into a message to staff that articulates the benefits to their team and the patients and families they are providing care. This effective communication is also essential to obtaining buy-in and motivating staff to engage in performing behaviors that support

T. K. Humbel (✉)
Clinical Nurse Manager, Baltimore, MD, USA

S. Bostic
Nurse Consultant, Upper Marlboro, MD, USA
e-mail: sharon@spbosticconsulting.com

R. Roberts-Turner, R. K. Shah (eds.), *Pocket Guide to Quality Improvement in Healthcare*,
https://doi.org/10.1007/978-3-030-70780-4_12

new processes and directives. The middle manager is a fundamental role within an organization to establish a productive and effective work environment for frontline staff in the clinical environment. According to Roussel and Swansburg [1], "a supportive climate produces clear communication and effective teamwork."

"Where the rubber meets the road" is ensuring effective teamwork is aimed to meet the needs of patients, families, and staff to obtain quality outcomes, and middle managers are adept at coordinating this action. Outcomes may be related to initiatives to improve patient care quality, patient satisfaction, staff satisfaction, etc. In a complex healthcare environment, middle managers rely on staff to drive quality outcomes and provide feedback to the team about performance. The result is a positive impact on unit and organizational goals that contribute to improvement efforts. These actions are usually nursing work performance behaviors such as patient education, pain assessments, and responding to patient requests. When staff members learn how their behavior makes a difference, they are motivated to contribute and seek opportunities to provide input to continuously improve other work-related processes to improve care and the work environment. For middle managers, eliciting input from staff and incorporating their ideas into patient care processes are important goals of effective communication.

Story

Earlier in the month, the organization underwent a printer and label upgrade for human milk labeling and identification. Claire is a bedside nurse who also functions as a charge nurse on her clinical unit. During a charge nurse meeting, Claire shared frustrations and concerns she has received from staff regarding the human milk labels not printing the appropriate patient information for patient identification outlined in the current policy. Also, Claire shared that not having all the necessary and vital patient information was disrupting the existing workflow by adding an extra step to verify the information as found on previously generated labels.

Discussions among the charge nurses identified the potential for unsafe workarounds that would ultimately risk the safety of the patient and facilitate unsafe work practices.

The unit manager communicated staff concerns during a system-level IT meeting. During this meeting it was discovered that due to the short implementation timeline, decisions from system-level leaders resulted in the approval and launch of the new printers and printer labels. The new technology was implemented without an understanding of the long-term effects or potential safety concerns. After an in-depth discussion, the same system-level leaders decided to reformat the human milk labels with input from the bedside staff to ensure the organizational policy was followed, and the potential for unsafe workarounds was mitigated.

In this situation, the lack of system-level communication and oversight of obtaining staff input and buy-in resulted in inefficiencies and potential safety concerns. Establishing forums to elicit feedback and facilitate open communication resulted in a change in structure and processes to support favorable outcomes.

Engagement and Trust

Engaging staff in quality improvement can be both challenging and rewarding. Capturing their enthusiasm to dive deep into the world of quality requires strategy and creativity fostered in a safe and trusting work culture. Keep in mind the importance of making quality improvement concepts relevant to their everyday practice being the key to engagement. As a middle-level manager, supporting scientific inquiry begins with a work culture that embraces a questioning attitude fueled by the "gut feeling" from frontline clinical staff. With those two elements in place, the spark to seek quality-based knowledge is ignited.

Each individual views the process and quality improvement differently. Individual perspective is shaped through knowledge, past work experiences, and interprofessional relationships in the work environment. Fostering continued professional growth and development is sustained in trusting relationships and ongoing engagement in the workplace.

Story 1

Rachel is a staff member on the night shift, and during a monthly staff meeting, she shared her concerns regarding the extended response times for families to receive return phone calls for patient updates. Even though she possessed no actual data to support her thoughts, it was a "gut feeling" that she had and one in which she was not isolated in her concerns. With support from her leadership team, parent rounds were conducted to validate or dispute the anecdotal feedback. With staff input, a survey of five questions were developed and asked of each parent and/or family member focusing specifically on response times for return phone calls.

After a week of meeting with the parents and families of the patients on the unit, the data revealed 48% of parents and families felt dissatisfied, and Rachel began to see the power of using a "gut feeling" to investigate further. In addition, her discussions with her manager revealed that along with the data she gathered of dissatisfied parents and families, it was important to know how the department rated in comparison with their competitors. With additional research and conversations with the quality director, they set a goal to decrease the rate of dissatisfied parents and families to below 10% which is lower than the average for the last 5 years.

With the small but powerful amount of data, Rachel sought guidance to initiate the next steps by taking her data and ideas to the unit-based shared governance council for open discussion. With support and mentorship from her unit manager, the spark to embark on a quality improvement journey was born.

Some of the most successful quality improvement initiatives are born from "gut feelings" that are further supported by collecting data and using tools such as key driver diagrams and PDSA cycles (Plan, Do, Study, Act) to develop a plan, set the work, and celebrate small wins. Having an overarching plan creates a shared mental model for stakeholders and is integral for success. As you continue to read the examples throughout this chapter, begin to reflect on how each example can be translated into your current work environment and among your staff members.

In the example above, the story captures the importance of engagement and the power of supporting the "gut feeling" of staff members. After all, they are at the point of care and functioning in an ever-changing environment. An important facet that goes hand in hand with engagement is trust. Establishing trusting relationships with staff will go a very long way, especially down the road of success, but with success also comes failure and mistrust. One of the most important lessons you can learn as a middle-level leader is that failures and negative feedback from staff and colleagues are not to be taken personally. Instead, one should look at suggestions for improvement as an opportunity for change and creative thinking to encourage others to adjust.

Middle managers can incorporate strategies to initiate trust by allowing opportunities for open and transparent feedback. According to Bramlett [2], each member of the staff is unique, and one's leadership style is customized to establish a trusting relationship. Trusting relationships can begin to be established through accountability, compassion, empathy, and approachability. When your staff feels that you have their best interest in mind and will advocate on their behalf, the foundations of a trusting relationship are established. An example of advocating on behalf of staff is below.

Story 2

Kathy started a new position and role on a fast-paced surgical trauma unit as the nurse manager. The initial 3 months were spent getting to know the staff, patient population, and surgeon teams. This is a high-performing, committed group of staff. One concern that Kathy heard repeatedly was related to workload. One issue brought forward by staff was that the only supply was in a storage room located at the far end of the nursing unit, and this was contributing to increased workload. This issue was resolved with suggestions directly from staff, who knew the problem and provided solutions. As middle manager, Kathy's role was to identify the resources and facilitate adding the additional supply room. Staff explained that the location of the storage room delayed their ability to obtain items needed for patient care or patient requests. This occurred within a large nursing unit with exceptionally large single-patient rooms. Staff members identified a smaller storage room on the opposite end of the nursing unit closer to patients' rooms that were farthest from the original supply room. Staff and Kathy worked directly with the central supply liaison to identify the most used supply items, secured shelving for the room, and in doing so, established a second storage room. This adjustment made a difference in the quality of patient care provided for patients and in the workload for the staff. Press Ganey top box scores for "nurse responsiveness to call bell" improved from 71% to 85% at the unit level. Kathy was able to implement a change with input from her staff, which helped to establish their trust and confidence in her as their new manager.

Accountability

Middle managers play a crucial role in fostering a culture that creates a strong partnership with their staff to provide safe and high quality of care to patients and families, supporting nurses' ability to practice to the highest level of their professional standards of nursing. "Personal accountability for ownership of the work implies an individual's obligation that demonstrates a personal connection to, and ownership of the principles and practices associated with the profession" [3]. This work culture should allow staff the opportunity to speak honestly and openly about work processes and practices and contribute to obtaining and sustaining improved outcomes. This culture, with a strong reverence to professional standards, helps to create a culture of ownership and accountability to team members, patients, and quality patient outcomes. Within the work environment emerges a culture where nurses accept personal accountability for their decisions, behaviors, actions, and the positive or negative impact on outcomes in the unit [3].

The middle manager is responsible for creating the space, time, and resources required for effective and meaningful work to evolve and occur. This may start as small as a unit-based team coming together to solve a practice or quality issue and may evolve into a formal shared governance or quality improvement committee or workgroup once the scope of the work is fully understood.

Story

Shelby is a senior staff member on a pediatric unit known for their increasing acuity and high practice standards. The unit is known for their high level of accountability to hold one another to high standards and use evidence-based practice to support safe and effective patient care outcomes. The manager on the unit is known for her supportive and transformational leadership style. This type of leadership style serves as the foundation of establishing a cohesive and robust unit culture. Supportive and transformational leadership fosters the process of goal setting, establishing fair and honest work ethics, showing appreciation for all levels of accomplishments, and creating a robust collaborative sense of teamwork. This effective leadership style results in a high level of accountability for the various levels of staff members in the department.

While receiving hand-off report from the night shift nurse, Shelby realized the bedside nurse was moving quickly through the hand-off report and missing integral elements to ensure safe care. As the bedside nurse was wrapping up the last of the handoff report, Shelby shared that before accepting care of the patients, they would need to review the orders and medication administration record (MAR). The night shift nurse became agitated, sharing that nothing in the orders and MAR has changed in the last 2 days. Also, the night shift RN stated that she had a rough night, was tired, and wanted to get home. Knowing that Shelby would be accountable for the patients once she accepted the handoff report, she stayed the course. She reminded the night shift nurse that she would not accept the care of the patient until they both reviewed the MAR, as stated in the routine of care guidelines.

Highly reliable organizations appreciate and enculturate systems thinking to ensure safe outcomes. The story above is a perfect example of the reluctance to simplify, one of the characteristics of a high reliable organization. Reluctance to simplify promotes people to reject the status quo by seeking to understand and embrace complex and dynamic thinking when seeking explanations [4]. Staff members who appreciate the reluctance to simplify hold their peers and colleagues accountable to high standards because they see the big picture and can foresee where safety risks may exist.

Continuous Quality Improvement (CQI) in Action

Middle managers are at the forefront of working with direct care staff who, at their best, are searching for new and innovative ways to provide quality care. The middle manager's role is to support a critical thinking environment to support staff's ability to develop and implement creative ideas that are evidence-based aimed to improve outcomes. Critical thinking skills must be grounded in the process, theory, and evidence-based practice. The middle manager is responsible for remaining abreast of best practices and current developments in their practice area. This may be accomplished through professional organization membership, accessing current evidence-based literature, and awareness of current trends in healthcare. The middle manager must learn how to value staff creativity, embrace vague ideas, establish collaborative relationships, as well as support staff in taking calculated risks in implementing improvements. Most importantly, the middle manager allows staff to fail and supports learning, growth and development, and the journey of improving outcomes [5].

Story

Nurses complained about the fast-paced nature of the postsurgical inpatient unit. They often experienced slow mornings with a low census and busy afternoons on the same day. This due to patients being admitted and returning from early morning surgery. Nurses became dissatisfied, and the unit's budget was impacted with increased salary and wages due to nurses leaving past the end of their shifts resulting in overtime. Staff complained about being unable to take lunch breaks, as well as the inability to leave work on time at the end of their shift.

The unit's shared governance decided to take on the challenge to address this issue, met a few times, and determined strategies to be implemented to resolve this issue. These strategies included enhancing time management competency for all nurses and implementing creative staffing patterns. The shared governance team determined that nurses could increase time management skills by beginning and documenting discharge teaching upon admission and supporting staff commitment to real-time documentation at the bedside. These changes allowed nurses to spend more time at the bedside with patients and families.

Mary collaborated with the staff to address this issue and determined the unit was able to change two vacant RN positions', work hours, and core job functions to address this need. These two nurses worked Monday to Friday from 1 pm to 9 pm. Two positions were created, approved, posted, and filled with two experienced nurses looking for a nontraditional schedule. Nurses filling these positions met the criteria for parking onsite, which was a benefit of the new positions. These positions met the needs of both day and night shift nursing teams. Nurses filling these positions were responsible for assisting with discharges, admissions during a shift change, break coverage, meeting coverage, and serving as a resource for novice staff members.

These changes increased staff satisfaction, as verbalized by nurses, with support for meal coverage, nurses being able to leave on time at the end of a shift, and support provided for staff recently off orientation. The unit experienced a significant increase in their NDNQI Press Ganey scores for the Practice Environment Scale subscale and Staffing and Resource Adequacy. The mean score for Staffing and Resource Adequacy improved by 2%, outperforming the unit and hospital mean scores. The two subscale questions with the most significant improvement included (1) adequate support services allow me to spend time with my patients and (2) enough staff to get the work done.

Mary, the nurse manager, also noted a reduction in salary expenses due to decreased extended shifts and overtime. Salary expenses for extended shifts by nurses decreased from an average of 220 hours ($6600) to 30 hours ($900) per pay period with an annual projected savings of $148,000. Mary generated reports in the timekeeping system in order to identify the few nurses who continued to have extended shifts and reach out to provide them targeted time management support so they could leave on time at the end of the shift.

Motivation

Middle managers should understand that the complexity of the healthcare environment results in an endless amount of work to be done. They also understand that frontline staff ultimately are the individuals who make the work happen. Once an opportunity for improvement is identified, a key indicator of success is the manager's ability to motivate staff, overcome resistance to change, and sustain the motivation and outcomes. Transparent communication, sharing of responsibilities, celebrating even the small wins, and sharing the workup and across the organization contribute to fueling motivation across all staff.

Fostering motivation takes time and assessment, and factors underlying motivation may vary from one person to the next. A customized approach requires creativity and out-of-the-box thinking. The use of rounding, providing real-time feedback, and identifying frontline champions are all tactics that can be used to boost motivation and sustain ongoing interest in quality improvement projects and initiatives.

Story

Grace and Karrie are both staff members of the same department. Grace serves as a shift leader, and Karrie has been a staff associate for a little more than a year and is just beginning to scratch the surface of showing confidence in her customer service skills. She also recently became more involved in department projects to increase customer satisfaction. During leader rounds, the manager and shift leader made purposeful touchpoints with both staff and patients to facilitate meaningful dialogue and face time. It was during these rounds that the manager stopped to compliment Karrie on her increased confidence level and the wonderful feedback she received about her communication style and compassionate personality. She found this the perfect opportunity to share her ideas about a particular infant swaddle blanket she felt was worth investing in based on her conversations with patients and the most recent literature she read about the importance of replicating a secure environment for newborns and infants.

Grace supported Karrie's idea and shared her thoughts and the feedback she received from customers sharing their dissatisfaction with traditional style receiving blankets and the difficulty parents have replicating the hospital-style swaddle. The manager recommended that Karrie and Grace lead a department initiative to critically assess the effectiveness of the current receiving blankets compared to the use of waffle blankets or muslin wraps now available in stores along with a cost comparison. With the full support and guidance from the unit manager, both Grace and Karrie were able to make contact with members from the purchasing to launch a trial in the department along with a cost analysis to present to other staff members and a small group of customers.

This example shows the importance of using a process to make meaningful touchpoints with staff to engage in conversations that relate to their everyday work. It also highlights the opportunity to allow staff to lead the work that will initiate change to improve outcomes. The motivating factor is the manager's guidance and ongoing support for staff to make a difference and be seen as a change agent.

Sustaining Improvement

The most effective method to sustain improvement is through making quality improvement a part of the daily routine or standard work and policies as appropriate. Managers want to avoid the perception that sustaining improvement is another task that is being added to their already busy day. After repetition, change of culture, and buy-in from staff, sustaining improvement can be put into "autopilot" mode that works on its own and only requires a spot check or recalibration at identified points in time.

The use of known sustainability models can be a helpful tool if you are looking for a more formal approach to sustainability. Still, simple tools such as performance boards, process control boards, and improvement huddles are just as effective. The above tools are used to help with keeping staff members informed of the work, progress, and successes. These tools also provide the opportunity to elicit involvement and feedback from others. As the middle manager, the responsibility is to provide support, ensure those who are affected by the change are engaged, serve as a resource to foster ongoing interest in quality improvement, as well as reward and recognize efforts. Middle managers engage staff in order to demonstrate that their work is valued, which allows staff to participate in decisions, leading to improved staff retention. Retaining high-performing, knowledgeable staff is vital in sustaining quality improvements.

Summary

The middle manager role is critical to an organization's success in implementing quality improvement changes and obtaining favorable outcomes. This individual, working closest with frontline staff, must possess skills in effective communication, leading change, overcoming obstacles and resistance, collaboration, and sustaining changes and outcomes. The middle manager role is critical in creating a flexible work culture, being open to new processes and technologies, committing to improving care for patients and families, and understanding the positive impact a positive work culture has on staff satisfaction and employee retention.

References

1. Roussel L, Swansburg R. Collaborative decision making and communication. In: Roussel L, editor. Management and leadership for nurse administrators. 6th ed. Burlington: Jones and Bartlett Learning; 2013. p. 178.

2. Bramlett C. Servant leadership roadmap. San Bernardino: Create Space Independent Publishing Platform; 2018. p. 71–5.
3. Porter-O'Grady T. Principles for sustaining shared/professional governance in nursing. Nurs Manag. 2019:31–41.
4. Agency for Healthcare Research and Quality. High reliability [Internet] 2019 Sep [cited 2020 Aug 15]. Available from: https://www.psnet.ahrq.gov/primer/high-reliability (2019).
5. Longo A. Change, complexity, and creativity. In: Roussel L, editor. Management and leadership for nurse administrators. Burlington: Jones and Bartlett Learning; 2013. p. 123–30.

Clinical Support Services' Crucial Role in Quality Improvement

13

Nikolas Mantasas

Introduction

Anyone working in healthcare – from executives to mid-level managers to frontline staff – knows that organizations today invest heavily in process improvement efforts. But frequently, these efforts fail to deliver on their objectives. In my 20 plus years in healthcare, I have encountered many detailed processes that appeared sound, but, in reality, they were flawed and ineffective. The problem often lies in developing and implementing processes without involving all parts of the organization. Sure, if you are a medical professional, a physician, a nurse, or a researcher, quality improvement (QI) principles have been a regular part of your training and experience, and you are likely skilled in assessing processes and making improvements to them along the way. However, as support services professionals know well, healthcare institutions do not consist solely of medical personnel or administrative staff with advanced degrees.

Critical to any operation is the staff in areas such as housekeeping, food and nutrition, and security. Medical and nursing staff in the operating room (OR), in intensive care units (ICUs), or the

N. Mantasas (✉)
Children's National Hospital, Washington, DC, USA
e-mail: NMANTASAS2@childrensnational.org

R. Roberts-Turner, R. K. Shah (eds.), *Pocket Guide to Quality Improvement in Healthcare*,
https://doi.org/10.1007/978-3-030-70780-4_13

emergency department (ED) may be skilled in evaluating and improving processes for their units, but what about the necessary processes that support medical and nursing staff? For instance, hauling waste out of the facility, or effectively cleaning and turning over rooms when a patient is discharged, or expediting food delivery to a patient in an inpatient unit? Who is responsible for improving these processes, and how do they go about it? Is the expectation that everyone understands statistical analysis or is six sigma black belt certified? One thing is certain: all processes, regardless of the department or work unit in a healthcare organization, can and should be improved. This obligation – to improve processes for our patients, families, guests, and employees – is shared by executives, management teams, and staff, alike, across an organization. I know that patients and families deserve it!

The fact that processes often are interrelated is another reason that we must consider nonmedical teams in our QI efforts. Waste and inefficiencies in one area have the potential to effect another in a significant way. Think of the patient discharge process as an example. We know that for a hospital to make room for a newly admitted patient, it must first complete the timely discharge of another patient. For timely discharge to occur, the medical team must write an order that is then implemented by the nursing team. In pediatric institutions, we often find that if discharges occur around mealtime, patients and families want to leave after the meal is served. The food and nutrition department becomes part of the process, and they must deliver the meal on time, if not early, so that the discharge is not delayed. Once the patient or family is discharged, housekeeping staff must respond quickly to clean the room and make it available for the next patient. These individual teams' processes are interconnected, and a gap or delay in one area has a negative impact on others downstream.

Any process is only as good as its weakest link. Medical and nursing teams may have efficient, tight processes, but once they rely on other departments to fulfill certain tasks, their hard work may be for naught. How do you get all processes to function smoothly? Your organization might be eager to educate all employees, including support services staff on statistical probabilities, central lines, upper and lower limits, tack times, and identifying kaizens. That may work well for some staff. But formal training programs may not be effective for many employees whose postsecondary education has focused on vocational, technical, or occupational training. Instead of delivering more training, one will need to take this complicated information and make it relevant to your audience.

We know from research that quality improvement is fundamental to an organization's overall success. We also know that in order to have a real impact and change the culture at all levels, we must focus holistically on every aspect of the business while engaging all employees in the effort. It is the only way you can change the culture to one that will always put quality and safety first to achieve the best possible outcomes for our patients.

In this chapter, we will explore this question: What is the best way to instill a quality improvement culture across all disciplines in a health system focusing on clinical support services?

The Journey

I learned about the importance of quality improvement in my first healthcare job as a clinical nutritionist working in the Lower East Side of Manhattan. I had just joined Rivington House, the nation's largest inpatient facility dedicated to the treatment of HIV/AIDS patients. It was 1997, and HIV/AIDS was still ravaging lives across the country. Patients, both male and female, often were admitted to Rivington House with a body mass index as low as 13 and an extremely poor prognosis – anything below 18.5 is considered underweight. I vividly remember one female patient, Liz, who was about 5 feet 6 inches tall and weighed only 60 pounds. She had lost so much muscle mass that she was severely contracted. In my role as a dietitian, I had to work closely with the nursing team, the physician, and the pharmacist on Liz's treatment plan. I was responsible for calculating the formulas for both intravenous nutrition and tube feedings and communicating that information to the rest of the clinical team. There needed to be a way that the clinical staff could supply nutrition to patients when the dietitians were off duty or busy with other patients. Liz had to receive nutrition as quickly as possible, and each patient had different needs. The pharmacist and I worked collaboratively to create a form that could be used to determine the exact recipe of nutrients that the nurses would supply to patients. It was a matter of plugging in the right information, and the formula could be calculated easily. We trained the clinical staff at Rivington House on how to use the form, which soon became an essential part of our operations. This new process demonstrated to the staff how one small change could make a big difference in care and outcomes.

As you consider how to instill a quality improvement culture in your organization, you will need to begin your journey by imparting a few concepts to your teams. The question is not whether to educate the staff on these critical topics, but how to go about it. No matter our level of education, most of us value knowledge, especially when we believe it will benefit us, produce better results, or make our work a little easier. How we acquire that knowledge can vary. For some, it requires the right environment – one that is supportive, nonjudgmental, and free of blame. It is worth spending the extra time and effort to create an environment that is conducive to your team's learning.

To help staff understand and use these concepts in their day-to-day tasks, you will want to provide clear and straightforward explanations. The staff will want to understand the reasons for the process, its components, and how to monitor it effectively to know that it is yielding the right results. One way to do that is to display progress measures prominently on QI boards in staff lounges and corridors (Fig. 13.1). These techniques will help you raise awareness and understanding of the concepts and give employees a greater sense of responsibility and accountability for QI. It is how you create an appetite for change to transform the culture. Healthcare leaders frequently believe that cultural transformation is a top-down initiative. It may start at the top, with the CEO or senior leadership team's vision, but culture takes shape at the frontline, where the employees interact with each other and with patients, families, and guests.

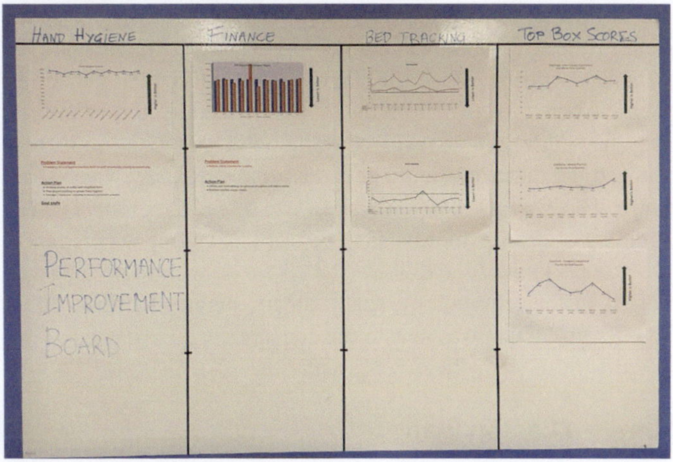

Fig. 13.1 Quality improvement board from the environmental services lounge at Children's National

Determine Baseline Knowledge

What is the best approach for teaching these concepts to housekeepers, food service staff, plumbers, electricians, and security officers? First, ensure the staff understands key terms. Team members must speak the same language. You need to perform a needs assessment to gauge a group's level of understanding. This can be done by asking questions at team huddles, meeting with union or group leaders, and meeting one-on-one with individuals. I would gather these responses and chart them on a whiteboard in my office. Despite a lack of training or formal education, the staff may be familiar with some of the concepts. Your assessment can help you determine how to tailor any instruction, where to provide general information, and where to give in-depth instruction.

Don't underestimate the staff – they will surprise you. One day last year, I was speaking with the housekeeping team about our organization's retirement plan. I was pleasantly surprised to learn that most of the staff had a good knowledge of investment terms, such as risk, future value, and compounding interest. This surprised me because the majority was not contributing to the plan. Although the knowledge was there and they understood the benefits, contributing to the plan was too difficult for many of them. After covering monthly bills and feeding their families, they had little left to save for retirement. This chat with them showed me that you should never assume you know what others know. This was also evident when we assessed the group's understanding of quality improvement theories and terms. As predicted, the group's knowledge followed a bell curve, with some staff well versed in the terminology, many others slightly familiar, and a smaller group that was new to the concepts.

Create a Lesson Plan

The next step is to develop a lesson plan to structure learning. Your plan should be clear and concise and not overwhelmed with jargon. As much as possible, it should include the use of colorful visuals and you can share by projector or LED monitor. Graphs, charts, photos, and illustrations are all helpful. Long verbal explanations of concepts and text-heavy slides are not. I have found that the best way to get a point across is to tell a story, especially when you make it relevant to the group's experience.

To explain to my staff why it was so important for the hospital to admit patients quickly, I relied on my own experience as a parent. We work in a children's hospital, and the majority of my staff are parents or grandparents. Some had used the hospital's services for their kids. It was apparent to me that this connection had to be leveraged. "Imagine that the patient who needs to be admitted is your child or grandchild," I began. "How would you feel about waiting forever in the emergency room or waiting room?"

Then I shared my personal account with the team. My son suffered from severe eczema when he was younger. During one bad flare-up, when we felt we had lost control of his care and treatment, we rushed him to the hospital where I was working at the time as the leader of support services. This is a highly respected institution in the community, and families travel from other parts of the state to bring their children there for care. I knew and trusted the caregivers there. My son's skin had become infected with staph, and as soon as the clinical team laid eyes on him, they told us he needed to be admitted for steroidal and antibiotic treatment. However, there were no inpatient beds available. So, we had to wait in the crowded emergency department for almost half the day.

When we finally arrived at the room and saw the admitting physician, she explained the treatment plan. Within 24 hours, he was doing much better and on his way to recovery. The wait had added to our anxiety. Housekeeping would come to my son's room twice daily, first in the morning to clean and then again in the afternoon to empty the waste bin and asked if we need any additional services. Everyone was very polite, but I knew that the processes were fragmented because whenever we asked for something, the time it took to respond to our request was inconsistent. An explanation was always given, but service varied depending on the time of day and service required. Food and nutrition responded promptly, but facilities took a while, or vice versa. A process cannot be effective if it is applied inconsistently.

I provided my feedback to the unit and emergency department nursing directors, both of whom I considered to be friends. Although I was nervous about sharing the feedback, I discovered that they actively listened to what I had to say without being defensive. They genuinely wanted constructive feedback.

I was careful, however, to begin with the positive parts of my experience. I had learned about the importance of starting with the positive from coaching exercises in the many different leadership development programs I had attended, including some facilitated by the Arbinger Group, Studer Group, Disney Institute, and the Ritz Carlton Customer Service Training. It was easy to share favorable feedback because the majority of our experience was excellent – for example, my son loved the food! While he wouldn't eat waffles at home, he gobbled up the ancient grain waffles they served. He adored the nurses and housekeepers, who were friendly, respectful, and very considerate of our privacy. They would always knock at the door and ask permission to enter. The physicians, nurses, and nurse assistants, alike, were patient and caring, and I knew they always had my son's well-being in mind.

With all that was going right at the hospital, they needed to fix a few processes to ensure these inconsistencies would not overshadow the team's great work.

Sharing stories with my staff helped as I use my stories to illustrate the point that the right processes can reduce the variability within an organization. The story brought the concepts home for the staff. They understood that it may be challenging when we are always asking them to make improvements – it's something our leadership focuses on constantly. The team now realizes that if we incorporate quality improvement and process improvement methodologies in everything we do, it will become part of our everyday work. When process improvement becomes a habit, a regular part of our work, it will be much easier to achieve our goals. When we get to zero surgical site infections, zero pressure injuries, zero readmissions, zero late trays, zero faulty lights, and zero soiled linen, we will know we have succeeded. All these zeros may one day translate to 100% patient satisfaction.

Patient satisfaction scores are receiving even more attention lately because of the way hospitals are reimbursed for care and now rewards or penalties are given to healthcare institutions based on their patient experience scores. Thus, improving patient satisfaction now also means improving an organization's reimbursement and its bottom line.

Educate in Real Time

Now that you have performed a needs assessment, identified gaps in knowledge, and established a plan, it's time to teach the material. You will want to present your content in a way that is interesting and easily understood.

Initially, you may have some short in-person sessions, but traditional classroom training does not work well for support services staff. Instead, seize on opportunities to explain QI concepts as they present themselves. Housekeeping staff who disinfect rooms every day know that despite a strong track record of properly cleaning rooms, there are occasional gaps. A patient may find breadcrumbs on a chair or debris in the shower drain. How were these things missed? I once posed this question to my staff: "How would you like to visit a hotel or a hospital and discover these items in your room when you arrived?" They agreed unanimously that they would be upset. So I asked, "How do we ensure that this does not happen here?" Someone in the group mentioned having a list of all the items that are supposed to be cleaned in the room. It was a great observation. "Is there such list, and if not, who will put it together?" Management? Not necessarily. Management can lead the conversation, but it's employees on the frontline who must provide input into the development of the checklist and any tool they will be using. They know patient rooms like the back of their hand and interact with patients and families daily. If you are a support services leader, your critical step here is not convincing your leader that you want staff input, it's persuading your frontline managers that the opinions of the staff are not just nice to have – they are essential. Your job is to get mid-level managers and supervisors on board and sharing in the belief that staff input and feedback is key. The wisdom of the crowd is far superior to the arrogance of one individual; I often solicit input from my managers and frontline employees, and they continue to exceed anything I could have conjured up by sitting behind a screen on my desk.

Another critical component of educating in real time is making sure your approach is inclusive of all staff – from all backgrounds, perspectives, and abilities. I once had the pleasure of working with a young man with special needs named Jonathan, who was part of our food and nutrition team, working with the dish cleaning crew. His responsibilities included testing the pH levels of cleaning solutions to ensure dishes were properly disinfected, and he needed to document the testing. Despite his developmental challenges, Jonathan was able to make the testing and documentation part of his regular routine because of the approach the team used to impart the concepts to him in real time. With Jonathan, we relied on systematic verbal reinforcement from department leaders and peers, as well as one-on-one conversations with his supervisor, Maria, with whom Jonathan had a special bond. She had taken him under her wing from his first day, and he trusted her. After about a month of message reinforcement, Jonathan had incorporated the pH testing and documenting into his routine. So when The Joint Commission reviewed our handwritten records, they asked to interview the employee whose name was on the logs. Jonathan shined, during the interview explaining in clear terms to the Joint Commission the importance of what he was testing and what he was documenting.

Checklists

Checklists are a great QI tool when designed carefully with input from staff and guidance from management. Once created, a checklist should be reassessed periodically to ensure it is still accurate. Processes change over time. Let's say, for example, if you add a new ultraviolet disinfection treatment to your room cleaning process, you'll need to add that step to your checklist. A checklist needs to be customized for a particular unit or area. Something that was designed for an inpatient unit might not work in cardiac care or perioperative areas.

Checklists are valuable as long as they are used. You can create the best list imaginable, but it won't matter if it's never operationalized. If the checklist isn't practical, it won't be used. Ultimately, staff is less likely to use a checklist they have not helped create. The more time you spend involving team members in a checklist's development, the more likely they'll put it to good use.

Make tools, like checklists, easily accessible. The language you use should be simple, and the tools should be shared at huddles, posted on boards, and made available electronically. When staff is on duty, helping patients on the floors, digital access is not always possible, so have laminated copies available. You can post laminated checklists in the kitchen, breakrooms, and on safety and quality boards. You can also place them on housekeeping carts. Consider color-coding items to make it easier to identify types of tasks at a glance. When it's a long checklist, with numerous steps, label critical steps in red and any optional or infrequently used steps in black.

Early in my career, I worked for a management firm that used checklists at every opportunity to conduct its business. That was great for those of us who were new to the company, but these same checklists became cumbersome for people who had been with the company a while. Their checklists were comprehensive, but often too long, and hampered efficiency. One organization I worked for had a nightly checklist for supervisors that included more than 40 items. Just completing the checklist occupied most of the shift, leaving little time for engaging with and supporting the staff. Evaluate your checklist frequently. Identify critical steps and eliminate duplications or unnecessary items. Your checklist should be a valuable tool, one that can even save lives – but it doesn't have to be onerous nor lengthy.

As the saying goes, a picture is worth a thousand words. Try to summarize your checklist steps using simple images instead of text. You'll notice, for example, that instructions for properly donning and doffing personal protective equipment invariably include images. During the COVID-19 pandemic, hospitals developed instructions with both still images and videos to ensure the procedures were clear to everyone. You can incorporate visuals into your checklists using icons.

Plan-Do-Study-Act

Another helpful device is the use of plan-do-study-act (PDSA) cycles. PDSA cycles allow you to try out (or practice) a chance to see how it will work (study it), should it be implemented broadly. Through the cycles, you can quickly learn about the likely success or potential failures of a planned change and use the process to modify your plan as needed. In our environmental services department, we struggled to get staff to return soiled microfiber mops for reprocessing. At the end of the day, soiled mops are deposited at a central location where our vendor would pick up the bins full of used mops, take them to a cleaning facility, and return them to our facility the following day. Thus, if 1000 mops were delivered that day, it stands to reason that 1000 mops would be returned the next. However, that never happened for us, and our inventory of clean mops diminished over time.

We decided to conduct a relatively easy PDSA cycle and followed our protocol of asking frontline staff (PLAN) for input. The employees appreciated being involved in the process. They identified a number of reasons why microfiber mops were not being returned. When the mops are distributed to staff at the beginning of the shift, they are dry and lightweight. Conversely, at the end of the day, the soiled mops are wet and heavy, not to mention messy. Unless we provided them with a simple, efficient way to return the mops to the point of collection, the staff found the task overly burdensome.

They asked if they could return soiled mop heads to a designated location on the floor where they worked instead of hauling them to the central location. Why couldn't we create a return point on every floor? There was only one way to find out if such a strategy could work: to add a collection bin at an agreed-upon location on each floor and have staff drop off their soiled mops at the end of each shift (DO). Collection bins were relocated, and staff instructed to bring soiled mops to the gathering point on the floor. Very quickly, we realized that staff were indeed bringing the mops to the new location, but rather than placing soiled mops in the bins, mops were discovered around the bins and on the floor (STUDY). We discovered that the collection bins had a small slot on top where mops were to be placed; the rest of the bin was locked. When we asked staff why the mops were not placed inside the bin properly, we discovered something interesting; soiled mops were collected in plastic bags, and the entire bag was brought to the soiled bin collection location. The bag full of mops did not fit through the slot. Frustrated and tired employees at the end of their shift, staff did not want to take the mops out one by one and place them in the bins. We could hardly blame them for not wanting the extra tasks that meant handling soiled mops again at the end of the shift. Moreover, this step likely constituted an infection control issue. The smart thing to do was to drop the entire bag of soiled mop heads next to the return bin.

We knew we had to improve the proposed process, which brings me to the last step (ACT). We continued to place the soiled return bins on the floors, but now we unlocked and opened the top of the bins, so the opening was more expansive, making it easier to drop the bags into the bins. This was a simple PDSA cycle that allowed us to plan, execute, assess, revise, and implement a new procedure in 48 hours. We could very quickly see if the new process worked, and if not, what additional changes needed to be made to help it succeed. The critical step here is timely feedback. There is no need to observe the process for days on end. Make some prompt observations, ask for quick suggestions from frontline staff, and proceed accordingly while continuing to observe and plan and implement the next steps.

Make Your Data Visible

Another step to successful QI is making the data available and visible to all. From the CEO to the housekeeper who cleans the nursing units, we all need access to the same data. Graphs and tables are prominently posted in our environmental services lounge. Data on bed turnaround minutes, hand hygiene, total operating expenses, supply costs, and patient and employee engagement scores are all posted in the department's QI board. The goal is for every member of the team to be able to understand the graphs and speak about the data. Not all employees can elaborate on every detail, but most are comfortable speaking about key points. All team members working in the inpatient nursing units, as well as our discharge team, can talk about the bed board and improvements we have made in turnaround times. Our storeroom clerk can speak about the steps taken to better control supplies and inventory. Other members that are regularly audited by infection control staff feel comfortable talking about hand hygiene or PPE utilization and processes.

It is critical that you also share the data and any metrics related to your team's progress with your leadership structure. Invite them to see the performance board displayed in the department and to share in your successes and setbacks. Better yet, have one of your frontline managers or staff discuss the team's latest efforts with them. These types of interactions provide an opportunity to not only impress your leaders but also promote and advance your staff. Successful organizations are the ones that can find and develop talent from within.

The QI message boards proved extremely useful during the COVID-19 pandemic. With social distancing measures in place, we could not conduct in-person huddles with the staff the way we had become accustomed to. The inability to not meet in person hindered the flow of information. Our education coordinator thought we could use the boards in the department to communicate COVID-19-related updates regularly. Any updates or news we wanted to share on COVID-19 data, processes, or procedures would be posted on the same board in the lounge. It became a one-stop shop for staff messages ranging from CEO announcements, to details on free Uber rides to work, to resources for mental health services. All this information was shared through the COVID-19 communication board and it became a permanent, invaluable tool.

Specialized Software

At Children's National Hospital, leaders have the opportunity to participate in a quality improvement program called QuILT (Quality Improvement Leadership Training). During the program, they learn about several useful QI tools and how to develop and track QI projects. They quickly discover that to track and improve processes, you must have good data. Without accurate and reliable data, you can't effectively track your progress, much less show an impact. As was mentioned earlier, the use of data is critical for QI tools, like PDSA cycles.

Tracking and analyzing trends such as patient throughput are essential for our department and especially support services departments. An analysis of throughput can show you how quickly patients are admitted, transferred, or discharged within the hospital. With so many patients admitted every day, and with a finite number of beds, it's vital that the process to admit and track new patients and patient flow be as smooth as possible. It can have an impact on your organization's reputation and financial performance. At Children's National, we tend to be at or close to capacity most of the year, which is usually a good problem for a healthcare system to have. This requires accurate, timely, and easily accessible data. Bed tracking applications can help, but not every organization has the luxury of investing in this type of software. For those that have it, the software provides a plethora of data, though some customization may be required to get to the specific information you need.

Good data can inform your decision of where to focus your efforts. After reviewing the data, our environmental services team identified that we needed to do a better job ensuring hospital rooms were cleaned soon after patients were discharged. It showed us we were not achieving national benchmarks. We launched a project to improve our room turnaround rate. The project required a process map and an intervention using LEAN principles. Process mapping was critical to understanding the sequence of events that occur from the time a patient is discharged to when the room is cleaned. As with any QI effort, there is a need for reliable data at each point in the process. We developed a process map to understand the flow of patients and resources and to uncover any gaps in the process. After a careful gap analysis and educating the team on the areas of concern, we were able to increase the percentage time that we responded to a vacated room within 60 minutes, from less than 50% to over 80% in 12 months. We eventually increased the goal to over 90%. Without access to reliable data, the project would never have gotten off the ground; we relied on input from frontline staff to uncover pain points and identify the reasons for delays in the process. Don't forget to use this opportunity to share your efforts and results not only with your direct leader but also with colleagues and leaders of other divisions, including the medical staff. After all, these improvements have organization-wide implications.

Pareto Charts

If you are undertaking an important process improvement project, you will need an executive sponsor. Typically, this happens early in the project's development. Without executive support, many projects fail, so it is an important consideration. If they approve of your proposals and plans, executive sponsors will champion your efforts with their peers, giving your project a greater chance for success. The use of data is one way to garner support from your executive sponsor and broader leadership team. Leaders use data to inform their vision and drive sustainable outcomes. Pareto charts can be very useful in bolstering your position or argument.

Looking at a multitude of numbers can be confusing for anyone trying to decipher meaning and develop insights. That's why it is important to take the time to create graphs and charts that make your point for you in a clear, visual way. Once you see a graph or some other visual representation of data, you often realize that the truth of the data is staring straight at you. I've often had epiphanies when seeing data displayed in a Pareto Chart.

A Pareto chart is a type of graph that includes both lines and bars that allows you to examine the frequency of events. Pareto charts are a simple way for a project to identify the most frequent defect, complaint, or another factor that can be categorized and quantified. At Children's National, we regularly use Pareto charts (Fig. 13.2) to illustrate relationships between variables and identify the "culprit" or problem area (i.e., where we should be focusing our attention). Pareto charts allow you to quickly show these relationships, and they are very effective when you are trying to steer a discussion or persuade leadership to approve a decision.

In one recent example, the senior leaders at Children's National were discussing employee injuries and the costs associated with them. They asked our team to research the problem and find some solutions. We knew that we needed to conduct a thorough analysis and provide accurate data. We also recognized it was essential to present the information to leadership in a way that helped them draw the right conclusions and make good decisions.

The problem centered on a recent uptick in the DART rate at Children's National. The DART (Days Away/Restricted or Job Transfer) rate is a calculation that describes the number of recordable employee incidents that resulted in days lost, restricted days, or transfers due to work-related injuries or illnesses. The first question here was "why was this happening?" and then "what can we do to address the problem?"

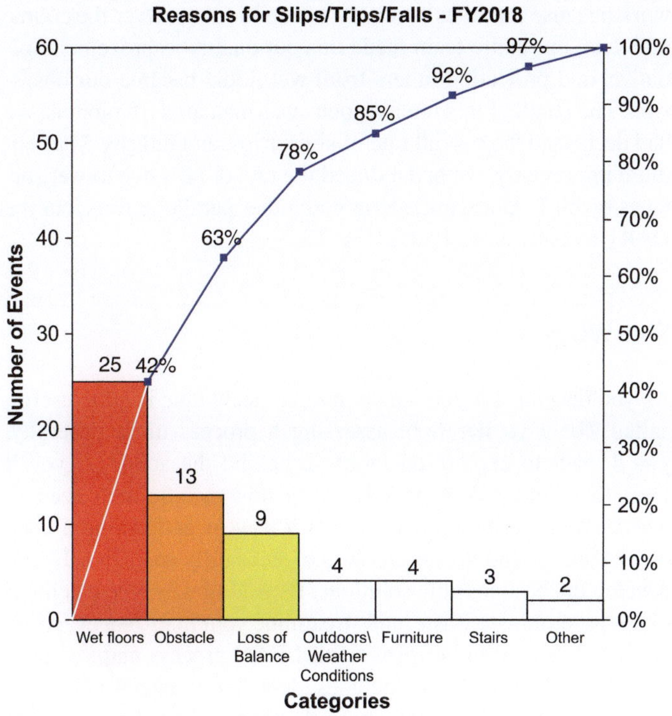

Fig. 13.2 Slips, trips, and falls Pareto chart

We needed data to learn more about the issue. With the help of a Pareto chart, we could determine where the defects might have occurred most often and where the organization should focus its resources. The data showed that the uptick in the DART rate was partially due to an increase in the number of employee slips, trips, and falls. We presented the data on the Pareto chart, showing the cost implications of the lost productivity, and we effectively convinced leadership that something had to be done.

We investigated further, digging deeper into the data to explore how the employee falls were taking place. Using a second Pareto chart, we showed that most slips, trips, and falls that resulted in lost productivity were due to wet floors (as opposed to objects in the pathways or staircases). This data point was crucial to our work because it told us precisely where to focus. Over the course of a year, our entire team made this our quality improvement initiative, and protecting others from wet floors became our obsession. The result of this intense focus was that, after 18 months, we had decreased the overall rate of slips, trips, and falls by 34%, but more importantly, we had reduced the rate of falls due to wet surfaces by 80%. Our work, along with other parallel efforts, cut the DART rates by almost 50% (Fig. 13.3).

Five Whys

As you develop a process map, another technique is quite useful, called *The Five Whys*. In assessing a process more generally, you'll want to explore the purpose behind the actions – you'll want to simply ask *why*. Why does this specific step need to occur? This questioning strategy is a way of performing a deep dive to understand the progression of steps fully and can help you develop the best possible solutions. By asking why, you can identify gaps, eliminate waste, and streamline your map. Not everyone is trained or able to perform a full LEAN process map, with its specific methodology that includes identifying kaizens and calculating tack times. Furthermore, in the teams I have led, everyone understands how to answer "why" and the importance of this line of questioning. However, asking "why" requires no formal training in a methodology. It can reveal where a process is broken or not function as intended. Questioning why must not be superficial. Don't just identify the first "why" that comes to mind; it might not lead to a solution. Instead, the team needs to continue asking "why" until a breakthrough in understanding is achieved. Management will not have all the solutions frontline employees hold the key. Involve them right away and carefully listen to their ideas and their complaints because within their pain points lies the potential opportunities to improve. You can pursue the "why" when conducting short PDSA cycles, but if you still haven't found your solution, don't despair. Keep trying a new PDSA cycle until you see results.

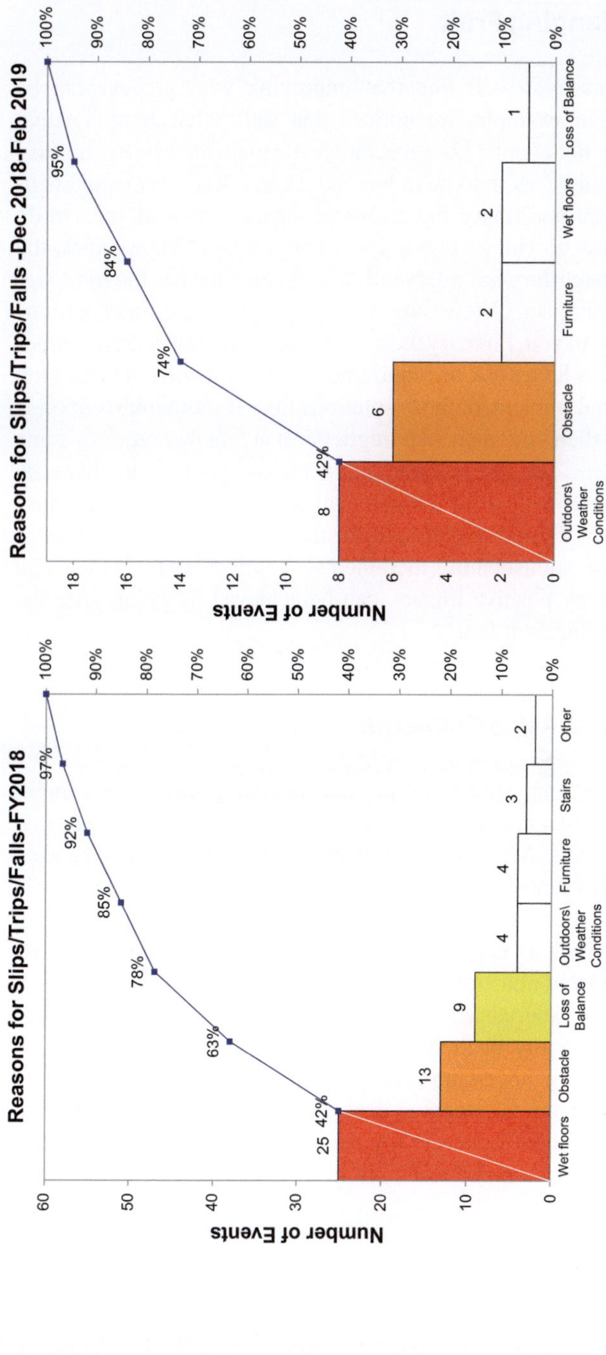

Fig. 13.3 Slips, trips, and falls Pareto chart showing progress

Low-Hanging Fruit

Sometimes you will find that improving your process can be costly. For example, we noticed that staff often complain that there are not enough housekeeping carts to do their jobs. The easy answer might seem to be to buy more carts. But what would happen if you don't have the resources (space, financial, etc.) to do that? How do you go about fixing the problem? Many times, the most straightforward intervention is the one that has the most significant impact. There are often many possible interventions available to you. First, try those that require limited or no resources but have a lesser ask or requirement – the so-called low-hanging fruit – and implement those solutions first. If more intervention is needed, then your next step might be an action that requires some investment. The last possible interventions are those that have the highest ask or require a significant amount of resources. Those should be left to the end, and for those steps, you'll likely need executive sponsorship. Incremental improvements, which can have a very positive impact, can be achieved by going after the low-hanging fruit first.

Stop and Ask a Colleague

There are times your frontline staff, including supervisors, might be met with a challenge they have not experienced before or that rarely occurs. Are there any just-in-time QI tools that can be used to support a positive outcome in these situations? The answer is yes. Whether it is related to an operating room team performing an operation, an emergency room team treating a trauma patient, or a food and nutrition team delivering a tray, team members will inevitably experience situations that they might not have encountered frequently in their careers. Or, it might be a situation in which there is uncertainty about how to proceed. What then? How do we prepare our teams to deal with the unexpected? These are the times where I instruct my team to pause and think critically about the situation or reach out to a colleague. When you are in doubt about your next steps, or experiencing a unique situation, ask a colleague and verify possible solutions before moving forward. Regardless of the situation, someone in your department or your organization likely has experienced something similar before. Reach out and ask for advice and confirm that your thinking on the matter is correct. Taking the time to pause and consult peers or other leaders is crucial here and a simple tool that can be beneficial not only in clinical settings but in hospital operations.

Conclusion

QI provides valuable tools to help support services teams make more reliable decisions on complex issues in healthcare. Simple QI tools can be used outside the clinical realm; however, it is important to remember that not everyone in healthcare is well versed in terminology or learns well in a highly academic setting. As healthcare professionals, we have the responsibility and obligation to teach all employees in our environment and provide them with the best tools so they can improve steps in any process, clinical or otherwise. As middle or frontline managers, we have an obligation to listen to our staff and hear their ideas, perspectives, and grievances. As executives, we should also listen, but expect in-depth analyses and thorough reviews and assessment. We should ask to see the data and require our management teams to use evidence to make improvements. Finally, we should trust and support our directors and managers to deliver results.

Processes can be complex, but leaders can simplify the concepts. In a healthy environment and under the right circumstances, leaders can teach all their support services staff simple QI concepts that can be used in everyday situations. Tools, such as PDSA cycles, QI boards with easy-to-understand data, asking *The Five Whys*, using Pareto charts, and pausing to ask a colleague for advice, can all help achieve the desired aim. Remember that all of our employees deserve continuous education that helps them improve. In fact, they are hungry for it. We owe it to them and to our patients and the community to keep learning and growing and to share our knowledge. A visit to your healthcare institution should be as smooth and safe as humanly possible, and that means preventing anything that can lead to hospital-acquired conditions and, at the same time, giving the patient the best possible experience. A focus on quality improvement can improve outcomes, enhance the patient experience, and reduce waste, thereby lowering healthcare costs. To achieve these results, however, QI must be embraced by all parts of the organization and at the higher levels of leadership. Then and only then will you see a profound impact on the entire healthcare system. It begins with the involvement of support services teams.

Pharmacy QI 101

14

Eric Manuel Balmir
and Fabienne L. Vastey

Pharmaceutical interventions are a cornerstone of modern-day medicine. Whether a patient is seen as an outpatient, inpatient, private practice, or emergency setting, the odds are that they will undoubtedly need some form of pharmacologic intervention to help improve their condition. Pharmacy has evolved through time where apothecarial concepts have become modernized through automation and technology. Such automation includes but is not limited to robotics and artificial intelligence. Pharmacy workflow and processes are currently performed with maximum precision at high speeds. Quality improvement in pharmacy is a delicate balance between efficiency and accuracy. In an attempt to understand pharmacy quality, one needs to understand the value of healthcare. Value-based care revolves around the idea of aligning all stakeholders of a system towards value delivered to patients [1]. Value according to the aforementioned definition increases in one of two ways, improving quality or decreasing cost. Cost is

E. M. Balmir (✉)
Children's National Hospital, Washington, DC, USA
e-mail: ebalmir@childrensnational.org

F. L. Vastey
New York-Presbyterian Brooklyn Methodist Hospital,
Brooklyn, NY, USA

R. Roberts-Turner, R. K. Shah (eds.), *Pocket Guide to Quality Improvement in Healthcare*,
https://doi.org/10.1007/978-3-030-70780-4_14

easy to comprehend when referring to value; it is most often associated with a service or item that is quantitative and tangible. Most often society correlates high quality to high cost. This is not necessarily always the case in healthcare. The focus of this chapter is to discuss some of the tenets of an effective pharmacy workflow designed to give the patient the best pharmaceutical care while accounting for cost restrictions.

Figure 14.1 shows the 12-step life cycle beginning with medication ordering and ending with charge capture. Although every step in the life cycle is important, this chapter's content specifically focuses on processes within the pharmacy department. These include procurement, storage, compounding, dispensing, and delivery processes within a hospital pharmacy setting. Pharmacy as a profession is designed to cure patients with ailments using pharmacologic interventions. Deviations in the life

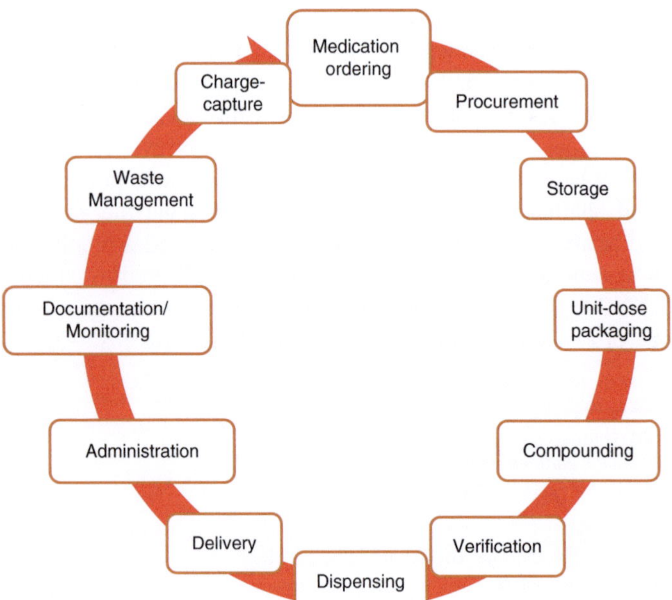

Fig. 14.1 Workflow of a medication order: the chart represents all steps involved in processing a medication order in a hospital setting

cycle can result in medication delays or may cause medication errors. In the United States, preventable medication errors or adverse events are the leading cause of death. Although many of our hospital systems have safeguards to avoid unintended outcomes, none of these safeguards are impenetrable. Automated solutions and clinical decision support systems are a couple of effective ways in reducing many types of errors. Figure 14.1 above highlights the 12 steps needed to effectively dispense ONE medication! Hypothetically, if an institution dispenses 1000 doses a day, this presents the hospital with 12,000 opportunities of making errors every day. Assuming a hospital is 99.99% accurate, the 0.01% error rate would still result in 1.2 errors a day which equals approximately 40 errors a month, still a very alarming number for an ideal institution. We are sure you would agree that this is not acceptable for your family member.

Procurement and Storage

Medication procurement is the act of purchasing and/or acquiring medications from a manufacturer or wholesaler. There are many variables that impact the success of having an effective procurement program at an organization. Drug shortages have become one of the biggest challenges in healthcare. The supply and demand ratios of medications have been the most impactful. Performance improvement as it relates to procuring and storing medications has several aspects to consider. There needs to be a system with an approving body to decide which medications to procure for a hospital. Pharmacies have to aim to buy medications at the lowest possible cost. Lastly, pharmacies must buy the correct amounts of medications and utilize them before the expiration date to minimize waste.

All hospitals in the United States have a Pharmacy and Therapeutics Committee (P&T Committee). This committee is a multidisciplinary team and is comprised of clinical providers, pharmacists, quality personnel, dieticians, and nurses. These individuals decide which medications the hospital will procure or add to formulary to support the needs of their patients. Medications placed on formulary are decided based on safety, effectiveness, and fiduciary responsibility. Once medications have been utilized for some time, it is important to measure the safety, clinical effectiveness, and financial status of the medication. This is most often achieved by one of two ways, completing a therapeutic class review (TCR) or conducting a medication use evaluation (MUE). TCRs are often conducted through various drug classes or similar medications which often treat the same ailments. An example of this is the nonsteroidal anti-inflammatory agents (NSAIDS) consisting of 12 different medications in this class. Some of the medications included in this class are ibuprofen, flurbiprofen, indomethacin, etc. Most hospitals would only carry a few of the drugs within this class. To carry all 12 NSAIDs would not be cost-effective. Conducting an MUE is the best way to determine which of the 12 medications an organization would carry. Similarly, when conducting an MUE, the following factors are considered in Fig. 14.2 [2].

Continuing with the medication use evaluation (MUE) process, an established timeframe is determined, and reports are extracted to make an assessment. The assessment includes provider names, specific patient care areas, cost, reimbursement, side effects, and inventory control. MUEs determine next steps for the medications allowing for novel medications in the same class to

Medication Use Evaluation (MUE) Factors
Patient Demographics
Drug Usage
Cost
Safety Events
Strengths Purchased/Dispensed
Side Effects
Reimbursement Profile

Fig. 14.2 Medication use evaluation (MUE) topics

replace old drugs or simply refine inventory allowing to maximize storage space and making sure only the most utilized strengths of the medications remain on the formulary and available on the shelf.

In relation to the procurement and storage process, physical inventory control plays a huge role in the day-to-day activity of a pharmacy. Once selected medications have been determined to be stocked at a hospital, the quantity and size of products are the next variables which have to be examined before evaluation of storage capacities. Utilizing tools like the therapeutic class review and medication use evaluation can help narrow down exactly what is needed for an institution to serve the needs of patient care. Most pharmacies do not have the luxury of having spacious storage facilities. Therefore, aspects such as size, storage conditions, and quantity determine how a purchasing team performs notating the real estate constraints of a pharmacy. Some pharmacies have turned to automation to help maximize purchasing performance. A hospital pharmacy is often faced with an extensive uncontrolled inventory when not managed effectively. A space-saving carousel storage system can organize, manage, and track medications maintaining effective inventory.

The success of utilizing a carousel system to track and maintain inventory is solely dependent on how often medications are counted accurately. This is with an assumed understanding that all employees working with the carousel understand the technology and concept of inventory management.

Accurate counts are the mainstays of an effective usage of a medication carousel. Although there are many advantages for procuring an automated dispensing cabinet (i.e., carousels) for maximizing storage capacity and minimizing footprint, there are some limitations. Only one operator can access the pharmaceutical inventory at a time. Vertical carousels are designed with an open matrix when selecting pharmaceuticals. Multiple drugs can be stacked on top of each other to maximize space. The end users can still have access to a number of medications at one time on the same drug shelf and can potentially select the wrong drug that may look alike or sound alike. Barcode technology is an essential component necessary to prevent making these types of picking errors. Carousels require many of the drugs to be prepackaged prior to loading the machine; a barcode scanning solution prior to the initial loading and dispensing process is essential.

Compounding and Dispensing

Let us give an example of the importance of compounding and dispensing. One early morning, the phone rings, and the overnight pharmacist who is usually calm and collected is hysterical this morning because she just realized she overdosed a 9-day-old baby in the neonatal intensive care unit (NICU). The pharmacist was supposed to dispense 41 mg/0.41 mL of drug for the baby and instead dispensed 140 mg/1.4 mL. Prior to administering the drug, the nurse double-checked the product. She realized the medication error and immediately called the pharmacist on duty. This is one of many compounding errors a pharmacist can make while inundated with work and understaffed. An event like this is what is considered a near-miss – the error never reached the patient. There are many safeguards one can consider to prevent such an error. In an organization where the patient population is mixed with adults and pediatrics, one may consider instituting a two-person independent check on all pediatric orders. Another safeguard can be segregating pediatric pharmacy personnel to a specific location or satellite, whereby the personnel are trained and accustomed to dosing pediatric patients.

Medication prescribing, preparation, compounding, and dispensing are complicated processes with several persons involved. In the pharmacy department, it starts with a procurement specialist, inventory coordinator, technicians, pharmacist, and delivery coordinators. In nursing, unit secretaries, medication coordinators, nurse techs, and finally nurses who administer the medications make up the personnel involved in the medication process. When a medication is ordered by a provider, it takes both pharmacy and nursing disciplines to collaborate to execute the order in a precise, timely manner.

In order to standardize how long a patient should wait for a medication after a physician has ordered it, the Centers for

Medicare and Medicaid Services (CMS) has provided time frames to hospitals such that healthcare workers can base workflows around meeting the required time for medication administration. A routine medication, meaning nonurgent, in a hospital setting, is expected to be administered to a patient 1–2 hours after the provider has prescribed it. A medication ordered with a frequency of STAT (an order which needs to be processed or administered immediately) has an expectation of being administered within 30 minutes of being prescribed by a provider. Failure to meet this 30-minute demand may have a negative impact on the patient. The anecdote below is an example of how a STAT medication delay was a factor in the demise of a child.

Hypothetically, imagine if you were to receive a call from a high-ranking healthcare professional like the chief operating officer of a hospital informing you there was a medication delay of over 4 hours involving an antibiotic for a critically ill patient. This medication delay was a result of the inability to locate the medication in the pharmacy for compounding. This can occur very easily in a busy hospital pharmacy. The sick child required immediate pharmaceutical intervention within 1 hour to reverse the deterioration. The medication was ordered appropriately by the provider; however due to several variables, the medication was not dispensed to the patient timely and contributed to the patient's decline. This unfortunate outcome would lead to a series of investigations (root cause analysis) in search of opportunities for workflow improvements within a pharmacy. These workflow improvements would identify bottlenecks which when resolved and would minimize negative outcomes. Medication delays are a major cause for serious adverse events. Delays can occur during any step of the medication use process from writing the order, verifying the order, compounding the medication, checking the ingredients, delivering the medication, and finally dispensing the prescribed medication. Delays in pharmacy are quite common no matter what the setting. This hypothetical example is one reason we embarked on a quality improvement initiative at our hospital examining medication times.

The success of executing a STAT medication timely is dependent on how well frontline workers communicate between all the steps. Communication is essential to drive, change, or maintain high productivity when multiple people are involved in executing the dispensing of medication in a timely fashion. Communication via data sharing is the most effective way to keep staff engaged and aware of turnaround time of STAT medications. Utilizing tools like key driver diagrams, control charts, and process map flows can facilitate performance improvement processes.

Figure 14.3 depicts a data control chart which plots the average time medication orders were reviewed by a pharmacist to the time the medication was delivered a week at a time. The graph shows the pharmacy department's turnaround time for a STAT medication that went from being greater than 110 minutes to less than 20 minutes over a year. The graph measures several variables: the gray-shaded areas represent the number of STAT medication orders that the department processed over 7 days. The plotted line indicates the average turnaround time each week for 1 year. There were three distinct centerline shifts in the graph indicating improvement in the department's turnaround time after three distinct process changes.

A quality improvement (QI) project ensued within the division of pharmacy where several inconsistencies were identified. Figure 14.4 Key Drivers and Key Interventions diagram outlined the QI project. The easiest intervention that had the most impact was the sharing of data via electronic mail to frontline staff. The amount of time that it took to process STAT medications was surprising to the pharmacy staff. Once the distribution of data was assigned to specific staff, there was more accountability in processing STAT orders. As represented by the first centerline shift in Fig. 14.3, the turnaround time for the department improved by 60%. The leadership team immediately educated the staff on the importance of a quicker turnaround time and enforced that a goal of less than 20 minutes' turnaround time per dose was a priority for the department. The leadership also impressed upon the staff on making sure safety was not compromised, and measuring safety events as a balancing measure was essential to the success of the project.

Assuming there is inventory available and readily accessible for personnel to execute a STAT order, the process should run

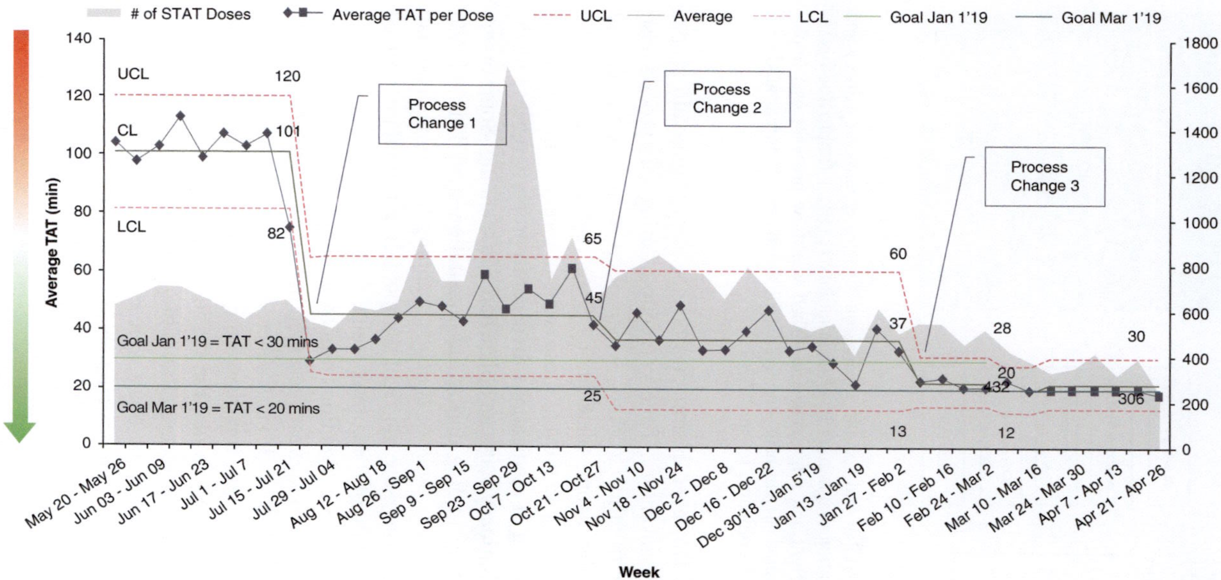

Fig. 14.3 Turnaround time for STAT medications over 1 year (x-chart). The red dashed line indicates the upper and lower control limits of turnaround time through a 12-month window, while the green solid line shows the target level from May 2019 through April 2020

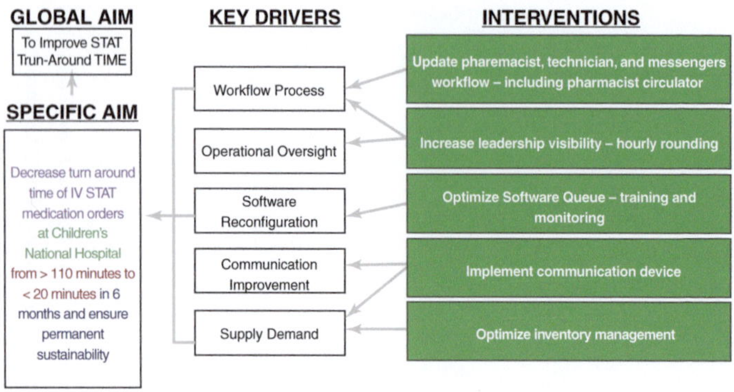

Fig. 14.4 Global and specific medication dispensing aims: key driver and key intervention diagram. A level of reliability (LOR) 1 (improving operational oversight and improving established workflow process) was implemented. Overall, department witnessed a 75% reduction in turnaround time by May 2020 compared to April 2019

smoothly. However, pharmacies do not always maintain proper medication inventory. Time perception during this process also differs for frontline workers, which often results in mistakes in selecting the wrong medications from rushing to process the orders. One way to prevent these types of errors is the use of barcode scanning of medications. In order to properly retrieve medications, pharmacy staff can utilize barcode scanning. Some orders require compounding during the preparation step. This can add more time to the process. Barcode scanning technology can also assist in making sure the right compounding formula is utilized for the selection of the correct recipe.

Some of the interventions needed to achieve goal in the pharmacy, in addition to those presented in Fig. 14.5, include:

To gauge how well staff adhered to all dispensing interventions, frequent usage reports were reviewed by operational managers. The reviews resulted in the identification of opportunities for increasing efficiency, eliminating problem elimination, and encouraging staff when goals were being met. Reports were further adjusted to detail specific shifts, individual employees, and different days of the week. The reports were also enhanced to

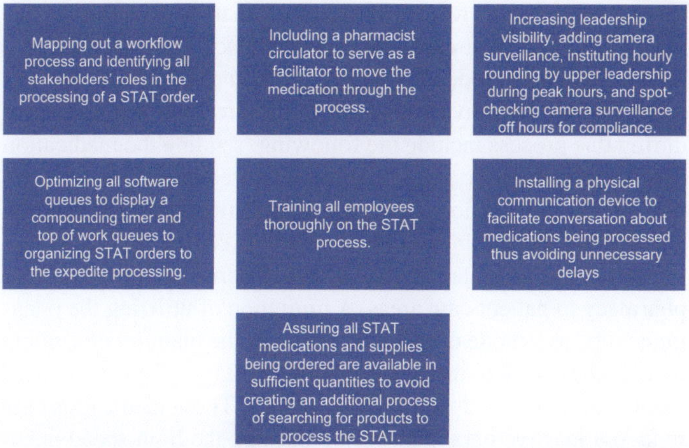

Fig. 14.5 Measurable interventions to achieve reduction in STAT turnaround time in a standard hospital pharmacy

include hospital census and total number of orders processed to account for downtime between STAT medication orders.

Delivery

A key component of pharmacy workflow is the delivery of medications. After proper medication verification, accurate preparation, and dispensing, the next course of action is to ensure that the correct medication is delivered to the right patient at the right time. Some of the many modes utilized for delivering medications to patients include pharmacy messengers, pneumatic tubes, or nursing personnel picking up medications for their assigned patients.

Although there are multiple modes of delivering medications, pneumatic tubes are sometimes the fastest way of getting medications directly to patient care areas. The process involves pharmacy staff obtaining the medication and scanning a barcode on the label or medication to track what time the medication was sent to the patient care areas. This requires communication and coordination for the caregiver to receive notification that the medication has arrived at the patient care unit. All pharmacy staff members are integral in each mode of delivery. Effective communication is imperative to the delivery process. Common errors that can occur during this process include the following: sending the medication to the wrong patient care area, spilling or breaking of medications during transport, or lodging of the medication carrier within the pneumatic tube within the system due to excessive weight.

Pneumatic tubes are not designed to carry all products from pharmacy to patient care areas. A limitation of utilizing the pneumatic tube as a mode of transport involves the inability of sending medications which require rigorous shaking of protein-based medications such as insulin or biologicals. These medications are rendered inactive once transported through the high-speed pneumatic tube as the proteins become denatured and ineffective. Hazardous medications, drugs greater than 500 mL (heavy), large containers, and drugs in large quantities require physical delivery to patient care areas. Some pharmacies have dedicated personnel to complete this task, sometimes referred to as "pharmacy messengers." Pharmacy messengers are often tasked to deliver medications directly to nurses if certain medications cannot be tubed or if they are urgently needed. The use of humans to transport medications is not error-free. This mode requires coordination and established processes such that nurses are always aware when medications arrive. In addition, nurses should also be aware of medications that are placed for retrieval on the patient care area. Commonly seen errors in this process include cases where medications are placed in the wrong patient's dedicated bin. This leads to nurses not being able to find the medication, hence, causing delay in administration of the medication.

In 2017, the Cleveland Clinic published an article "Nursing and Pharmacy Team Up to Improve Medication Delivery Process." The article highlighted that interdisciplinary collaboration is essential in dissecting workflow processes in efforts to change common perception and common practices when faced with adversity.

Controlled substances require tracking and tracing to establish a chain of custody often times requiring signature, return, and receipts of delivery. Most organizations mandate licensed nurses to pick up controlled medications for their individual patients. Errors that can occur during this process include handing over the wrong medication to the nurse; the nurse may not recognize that he or she has received the wrong medication and eventually administer the wrong medication to the patient. There have been real-life scenarios where this has occurred. The standard prior to any medication administration is using two patient identifiers, such as patient name and medical record number or date of birth.

It has been widely established that some medications require immediate delivery after preparation due to the instability of the drug. Many injectable medications need to be freshly prepared to ensure product integrity by maximizing drug stability duration. Ampicillin is a highly effective antibiotic used for treating a wide array of bacterial infections that when prepared for intravenous administration has a stability period of 60 minutes [3]. Imagine a scenario where a pharmacy has in-stock a properly procured and stored batch of ampicillin powder for dilution. A patient who weighs roughly 100 pounds develops a gastrointestinal tract infection, and her physician upon consultation with a pharmacist properly places an order for ampicillin 500 mg to be immediately administered to the patient and repeated every 6 hours. The medication order is prepared and verified by a pharmacist and ready to leave the pharmacy. Medications such as ampicillin, with short stability, require immediate delivery and coordination with the administering nurse to ensure the medication is administered while the ingredients are still active. Careful timing has to be considered to assure the integrity of the product prior to administering. The American Society of Health-System Pharmacists (ASHP), the body responsible for creating the minimum standards/requirements for hospital pharmacies, recommends a continuous thorough evaluation of delivery methods as this step is associated with huge potentials/platforms for medication errors to occur [4].

One way that pharmacies have been able to streamline their process is through the utilization of color-coded bin systems. The colors utilized in this bin system are similar to the traffic light. In this system, red means stop and check, yellow means hold/pause, and green means checked by pharmacist and ready to go. Additionally, the bins are labeled with the color of the bins in order to accommodate employees who may be colorblind. Regardless of the layout of a pharmacy, the traffic light bin labeling method facilitates workflow by assuring that only checked medications in the green bins are dispensed.

The American Society of Health-System Pharmacists (ASHP), the body responsible for creating the minimum standards/requirements for hospital pharmacies, recommends a continuous thorough evaluation of delivery methods as this step is associated with huge potentials/platforms for medication errors to occur [5].

Quality Control

Quality control is an aspect of pharmacy that is necessary and essential. Due to the complexity of the medication process, healthcare providers involved in the management of medications are known to make medication errors. To put this in perspective, one must understand the Swiss Cheese Model. The Swiss Cheese Model in pharmacy is a series of barriers in place to prevent a medication error. Each step, as shown in Fig. 14.6, represents a slice of cheese with gaps in our medication management process.

This is a dynamic process, and each hole size changes with each medication ordering scenario. When the holes align, a breakdown in our safeguard process occurs, and a preventable error is

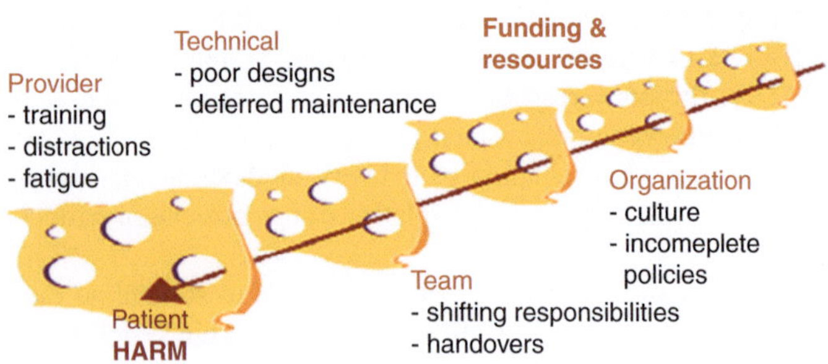

Fig. 14.6 Swiss Cheese Model in healthcare [6]

inevitable. Medication errors, although frequent, are just one aspect of medical errors in the hospital setting. However, not all the medication errors lead to actual harm. An error is defined as the failure of a planned action to be completed as intended (i.e., error of execution) or the use of a wrong plan to achieve an aim (i.e., error of planning) [7].

Managing medications face a wide array of challenges, from serving the needs of increasing populations to managing supply and demand issues. Safeguards that are put in place to mitigate errors will forever remain a professional challenge as new healthcare providers enter the system. Ultimately, pharmacies share a common goal which is to improve care through robust, high reliable quality improvement programs.

A pharmacy must have a system to manage and categorize the severity of errors. One example of such system is depicted in Fig. 14.7.

Figure 14.7 presents nine categories for categorizing medication errors as established by the National Coordinating Council for Medication Error Reporting and Prevention (NCC MERP) Index. NCC MERP is an independent organization responsible for addressing causes of medication errors and promoting the practices to ensure increased safe use of medications. Medication safety must be every pharmacy's top priority. One may think no process is perfect and medication errors are inevitable; however, quality controls need to be established where all errors are reviewed, tracked, and trended to identify system issues to prevent future errors from occurring. One way to measure medication errors is to look at the severity of the error. The error grading system ranges from A to I. An "A or B" grade error is most desirable as this error is termed a near-miss and never reach the patient. A grade "C" error reaches the patient, but does not cause any harm (see red man displayed in Fig. 14.8). Grades D and E are errors where monitoring is required to determine if a patient has experienced any harm from the error. Lastly, errors graded F through I not only reach the patient but can cause temporary to permanent harm up to death.

As presented in Fig. 14.7, National Coordinating Council for Medication Error Reporting and Prevention Index, each slice in

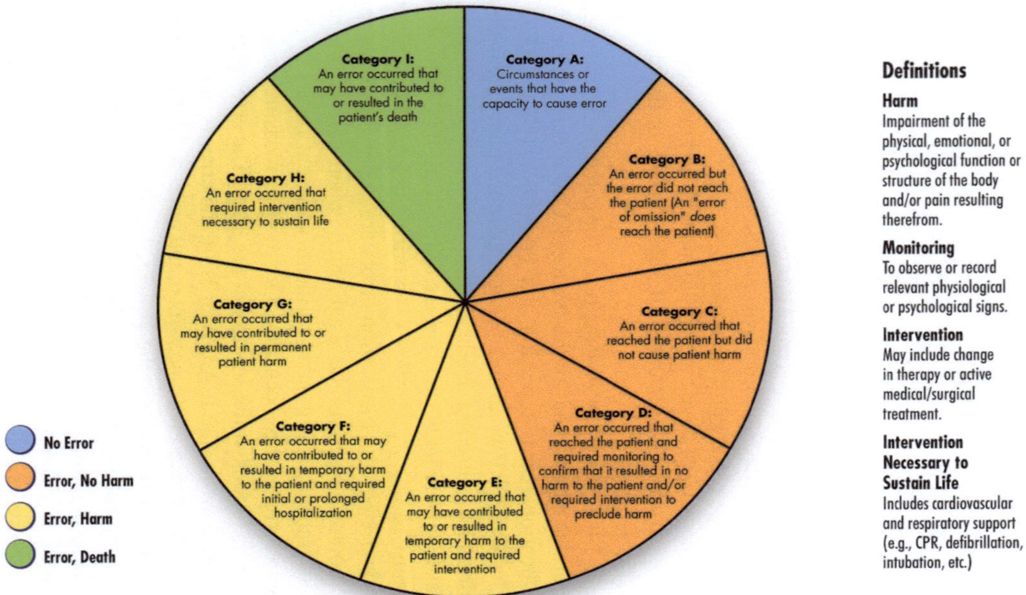

Fig. 14.7 National Coordinating Council for Medication Error Reporting and Prevention Index. (© 2001 National Coordinating Council for Medication Error Reporting and Prevention. All Rights Reserved)

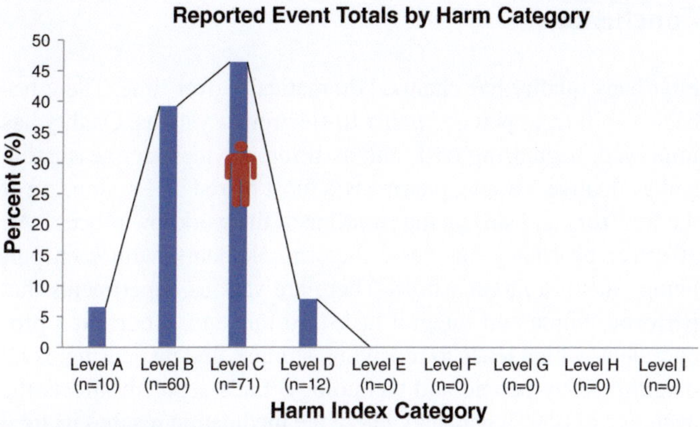

Fig. 14.8 Monthly snapshot of reported events totals by harm category: This figure represents a hospital with a strong patient safety culture

the pie is depicted by a color. Each color denotes the severity of an error: blue, no error; orange, error no harm; yellow, error with harm, and lastly green, error causing death [8].

An organization with a strong patient safety culture should have many reported near-misses (Grade A errors). A sample snapshot of a hypothetical monthly report is represented in Fig. 14.8. The figure depicts what the severity chart can look like when one properly evaluates its quality control metrics and can easily be shared with leadership with the person symbol representing level C and above where the errors reach the patients.

Of the 153 medication errors exemplified above, 45% of the errors reached the patient but caused no harm, and 55% of the errors were caught prior to reaching the patient. The hypothetical institution had no event that resulted in any sort of temporary or permanent harm to patient. Most importantly, no deaths occurred as a result of any medication error. This is a standardized manner to convey, at a very high level, many facets about the pharmacy process and is easy to interpret for myriad audiences.

Conclusion

Pharmacy quality has changed dramatically over time. There has been a shift from pen and paper to electronic systems. Quality has improved, decreasing cost, and assuring services are measurable and evaluative. People, pharmacy's most prized possession, are at the forefront and still on the frontline of the workflow process. An effective pharmacy has basic factorial elements, with each part being part of a larger whole. There are various departments that perform unique and integral tasks. To this end, medication procurement, which leads to receiving, storage, and dispensing, is all determined by people and technology. Each segment affects the accuracy of how, when, and where the medication reaches its final destination. Overall, the ultimate goal of the workflow process is patients receiving accurate medication in a timely and cost-effective manner. Finally, when the patient receives successful pharmaceutical care, our hope is that quality is the underlying factor, which is sometimes evident but not always apparent. The balance of efficiency and accuracy is always present in our pursuit in effective patient care. Patient safety will always remain the top priority.

References

1. Global coalition for value in health care, World Economic Forum Shaping the future of health, weforum.org/project/value in healthcare.
2. Nursing and Pharmacy Team Up to Improve Medication Delivery Process. Consult QD. https://consultqd.clevelandclinic.org/nursing-pharmacy-team-improve-medication-delivery-process. Published 2020. Accessed 29 May 2020.
3. American Society of Health-System Pharmacists. ASHP guidelines on medication-use evaluation. Am J Health-Syst Pharm. 1996;53:1953–5.
4. Ampicillin for injection [package insert]. New York: Pfizer Pharmaceuticals Inc; 2010.
5. Mazur LM, Chen S. Understanding and reducing the medication delivery waste via systems mapping and analysis. Health Care Manage Sci. 2008;11:55–65. https://doi.org/10.1007/s10729-007-9024-9.

6. American Society of Health-System Pharmacists. ASHP guidelines on the safe use of automated dispensing devices. Am J Health-Syst Pharm. 2010;67:483–90.
7. Reason JT. Human Error. Cambridge: Cambridge University Press; 1990.
8. Categories of Medication Error Classification. Content last reviewed. Agency for Healthcare Research and Quality, Rockville; August 2012. https://www.ahrq.gov/patient-safety/resources/match/matchtab6.html

15 What Hospital Board Members Should Ask About Quality and Safety

Sandip A. Godambe, Robert C. Lloyd, Maya S. Godambe, and Stephanie Borinsky

Chapter Objectives

1. To understand the role of the health system board in driving quality and safety as a business strategy
2. To understand the reasons behind the global focus on healthcare quality
3. To understand the concept of high reliability

S. A. Godambe (✉)
Department of Quality and Safety and Division of Pediatric Emergency Medicine, Children's Hospital of The King's Daughters Health System, Norfolk, VA, USA

Department of Pediatrics, Eastern Virginia Medical School, Norfolk, VA, USA
e-mail: Sandip.Godambe@chkd.org

R. C. Lloyd
Institute of Healthcare Improvement, Boston, MA, USA
e-mail: rlloyd@ihi.org

M. S. Godambe · S. Borinsky
Department of Pediatrics, Eastern Virginia Medical School, Norfolk, VA, USA
e-mail: mgodambe@gmu.edu; stephanie.borinsky@chkd.org

R. Roberts-Turner, R. K. Shah (eds.), *Pocket Guide to Quality Improvement in Healthcare*,
https://doi.org/10.1007/978-3-030-70780-4_15

4. To understand the aspects of quality that matter to our patients
5. To understand the Baldrige approach to evaluating processes and outcomes
6. To be able to apply Deming's System of Profound Knowledge (SOPK) to any quality improvement project
7. To be able to explain and apply the IHI Model for Improvement
8. To understand how to interpret statistical process control (SPC) charts
9. To understand the value of organizational celebration in healthcare settings

The Question?

Why did you agree to be a board member? This is a simple question but one that receives a wide variety of responses. Some answers are rather vague and reference things such as "fulfilling our mission and vision." Others refer to "demonstrating our values." Still others get a little more specific and cite things, such as "improve market share," "maintain financial viability," "be rated as 'excellent' by external reviewers," or "be recognized as the employer of choice in our area." While useful, the problem with all of these responses is that they miss the singularly most important response, which allows an organization to excel. The simple answer for achieving excellence is "to make quality our central business strategy."

Dr. W. Edwards Deming, one of the founders of the modern quality movement, provided board members, senior leaders, and managers with guidance on how to make quality the central focus of the organization. In his two classic books (*Out of the Crisis, 1992* [1] and *The New Economics, 1994* [2]) and in his consultations with leaders, he offered short provocations:

- What business are you in?
- By what method do you plan to experience improvement?
- Who is responsible for quality?

- Quality is determined by the top management. It cannot be delegated.
- Where is quality made? The answer is by the top management. The quality of the output of a company cannot be better than the quality determined at the top.

In addition to offering challenging provocations, however, he also offered practical guidance on how quality should fit into an organization's strategic plan. This is best captured by what has become known as the Deming chain reaction shown in Fig. 15.1. This diagram grew out of Dr. Deming's work with the Union of Japanese Scientists and Engineers in the 1950s. According to Deming [1], "This chain reaction was on the blackboard of every meeting with top management in Japan from July 1950 onward."

What is blatantly clear in this chain reaction is that it begins with quality not with "hitting performance or financial targets." This sequence shows the logical consequences of transforming management and making quality the organization's overarching strategy for the long run.

Although the chain reaction notion provides a good starting point to think about the logical sequence of events required for an organization to stay in business and add value to society, what is

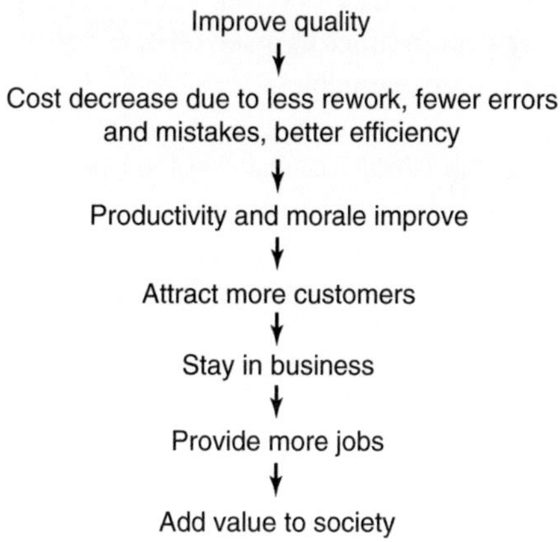
Improve quality
Cost decrease due to less rework, fewer errors and mistakes, better efficiency
Productivity and morale improve
Attract more customers
Stay in business
Provide more jobs
Add value to society

Fig. 15.1 Adaptation of Deming's chain reaction. (Source: Lloyd [3], 2nd ed., 332. Used with permission from the Deming Institute)

needed is a way to move beyond a conceptual model and evaluate the specific activities and behaviors that leaders need to support to make quality their central business strategy. In 1985, such a framework began to emerge. Members of Associates in Process Improvement (API) began to develop a template designed to help leaders incorporate the philosophy and concepts taught by Dr. Deming into the way they managed their organizations. In 1987, they formalized this framework and named it Quality as a Business Strategy (QBS). The three basic principles behind its development are that an organization needs to:

1. Establish a foundation of continuously matching products and services to a defined need of the organization and its customers through the design and redesign of processes, products, and services.
2. Perform as a system to achieve this matching of products and services with the defined needs as the targets or goals of the organization.
3. Maintain a set of methods to ensure that changes result in real improvements to the organization.

The details behind QBS can be found in the publication *Quality as a Business Strategy* [4]. In this and their other related publications [5, 6], they describe the five activities that leaders need to carry out in order to make QBS a reality. The five QBS activities for leaders include:

1. Establishing constancy of purpose in the organization (mission, vision, and values)
2. Understanding the organization as a system
3. Designing and managing a system for gathering information for improvement
4. Conducting planning for improvement and integrating it with business planning
5. Managing and learning from a portfolio of improvement initiatives

These five activities can be traced back directly to Dr. Deming's classic chain reaction and his focus on why leaders need to view their organization as a system with many interrelated processes. By having a singular focus on quality, all the other links in the chain reaction become apparent.

The Challenge

Population health, Plan-Do-Study-Act (PDSA), clinically integrated networks (CINs), Model for Improvement, Lean, Six Sigma, ISO, the jargon involved in addressing healthcare quality improvement can be overwhelming and a little foreign to many who are not trained in the science of improvement. When leaders share data slides at board meetings, they can unknowingly create a barrier to sharing their information with, and receiving feedback from, capable and engaged board members. These same members may be unwilling to challenge the status quo with seemingly irrelevant questions when the sheer overabundance of data falsely gives the impression that all is well. Furthermore, if management is presenting data in the aggregate (comparing this month's average to last month's average, the average this quarter to the same quarter a year ago, or rating and ranking performance indicators with the use of red/yellow/green graphics), not only will it convey the wrong impressions but also hinder opportunities for lasting improvement. So, what questions should board members be asking?

The Foundation for Quality

In 1999, *To Err Is Human* [7] was published by the Institute of Medicine (IOM), highlighting the unnecessary harm that was resulting from inefficiencies and gaps in our healthcare system structures and processes. Over the ensuing 20 years, a clearer focus on quality improvement and safety science has emerged. Three decades ago, quality and safety improvement projects in health and social service industries were novel or nonexistent. Now, the lay public expects continuous process improvement to be part of any health system's daily operations. Dr. W. Edwards

Deming showed, through his chain reaction concept, that when an organization in any sector focuses on improving quality, the end result is organizational success, quantified by more business and the need for more employees [2]. Dr. Richard Brilli, quality pioneer and former chief medical officer at Nationwide Children's Hospital, and others have long said that "*Quality is not extra work. It is the work*" (personal communication). Not surprisingly, hospital boards are expected to have statutory oversight for the comprehensive quality and safety of the care provided by their health system. In this chapter, we will provide an introduction of key quality improvement principles that all board members should understand in order to be effective in their role. **The "Points to Ponder" boxes in this chapter represent potential questions any board member should ask an improvement team member or leader.**

Achievement of both internal and external performance expectations cannot be achieved by studying aggregated data and summary statistics. Manufacturing industries have demonstrated this principle for decades. While there are quarterly summaries that are used to show how a company is doing in the aggregate, behind these summaries are detailed charts maintained by staff and managers that are aimed at diagnosing the variation in their processes hour by hour and day by day. Healthcare board members, therefore, need to switch their mindsets to begin looking at data from a quality improvement perspective, not from an aggregated perspective. Board training and development on how to adapt and spread a new mindset is essential if new levels of performance are desired. Hospital walk rounds on frontline team member activities, first-hand sharing of patient stories at board meetings, shadowing clinicians in their daily patient care activities, interacting with patient-family advisory council members, and other direct interactions with daily hospital operations are only a few examples of how board members have gained valuable insights about organizational performance [8].

In summary, the drive for improvement needs to come from an intrinsic will to want to improve. Building continuous improvement into an organizational culture can be challenging, but organizations that have successfully achieved this have flourished and endured. Their patients and their families, team members, and communities, all benefit when the organization has constancy of purpose and makes quality their central business strategy. Identification of opportunities for improvement, with resulting solutions through structured problem-solving by frontline team members, occurs routinely in such organizations. These ideas are vetted, and appropriate resources (i.e., time to work on improvement, as well as staffing and monetary resources) are provided when necessary, to ensure their success. Connecting outcomes, safety issues, patient and family needs, and organizational priorities with organizational capability and capacity for improvement can be facilitated or hindered by a hospital board. A shift from a reactive, quality assurance or firefighting approach to quality and safety to a proactive and planned approach, aligned with high-reliability organizational principles, lights the pathway to success.

Creating High-Reliability Organizations

Healthcare organizations are being pressured to continuously improve the safety and reliability of their processes and systems. Boards are being held accountable for making sure that safety and reliability are an inherent part of the organization's culture and operations. Yet, the healthcare industry is one of the most error-prone industries in existence today. The Institute of Medicine (IOM) in 1999 highlighted key issues with safety in healthcare settings in its seminal report, *To Err Is Human: Building a Safer Health System* [7]. This was followed by the second IOM report, *Crossing the Quality Chasm* [9], in 2001. A central theme in these reports is that healthcare organizations need to become high-reliability organizations (HROs).

Reliability refers to the ability of a system to repeatedly produce a quality product or safely deliver a service, with minimal variation. Its applicability to safety and value-based healthcare is self-evident. Nonetheless, the attainment of HRO principles can be challenging given the complexity of healthcare organizations and the desire on the part of many practitioners for total autonomy in making clinical decisions. On the contrary, building standardized reliable systems does not mean the loss of autonomy [3]. Weick and Sutcliffe [10] best described HROs as "operating continuously under trying conditions and having fewer than their fair share of major incidents." Examples of HROs are the airline industry, US Navy aircraft carriers and submarines, and the nuclear industry. These industries create "mindful infrastructures" that track unexpected events, no matter the magnitude, and assess their impact on reliable performance. They do this by tracking even minute failures, resisting oversimplification of the explanation, building a strong culture of situational awareness, remaining sensitive to operations, building and maintaining capabilities for resilience when bad outcomes or events occur, and taking advantage of expertise, no matter where the location is, to create timely solutions that prevent recurrence of adverse events and errors.

HRO Frameworks

The F-O-R-C-E mnemonic is used at Children's Hospital of The King's Daughters (CHKD) to remember the HRO principles (Fig. 15.2). The first three HRO principles refer to behaviors related to anticipating a safety event in order to prevent their occurrence. The last two principles apply after a safety event has

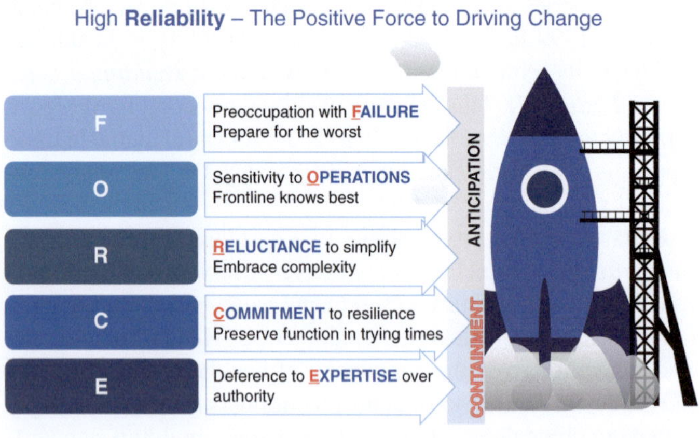

Fig. 15.2 Frontline. (Figure created by S. Godambe; template for figure provided by and used with permission from PresenterMedia.com)

occurred to contain the event. As an example, an imaginary hospital system, known as the world's most reliable hospital, located in Anywhereville, USA, had been tracking patient falls on a run chart (which will be explained later in this chapter). They have noticed an upward statistical trend in the number of falls which, fortunately, resulted in no injuries. However, there were concerns that a fall with significant patient injury could result if the reasons for this upward trend were not addressed. Within several hours of recognizing the data trend, the organization's leadership team commissioned a workgroup to conduct a root cause analysis (RCA) and determine why the falls were increasing. The trend on the run chart was clear evidence that this was not "normal variation." However, there was no clear explanation from the local unit leaders for the increase in falls. These actions represented a lack of focus on a "preoccupation with failure" and a "reluctance to simplify" existing processes.

The workgroup then engaged all frontline stakeholders, understanding the importance of "sensitivity to operations" and "deference to expertise." The organization's "commitment to resilience," through their rapid and timely investigation of these events, revealed that the organization had recently changed to a newer and less costly floor cleaner, which had increased soap content and dry time. Through structured problem-solving and rapid-cycle testing using PDSA cycles (to be discussed later in this chapter), both the new cleaner and the fact that the socks given to patients did not have rubber strips on the bottom to increase traction on the floor were felt to be responsible for the increase in minor patient falls. After the change back to the original cleaner and implementation of new socks with rubber strips, the frequency of falls declined to zero. HRO-related questions should be entertained whenever safety events are discussed at board meetings.

Points to Ponder

- What is being done to prevent a harm event from recurring at our organization?
- Are systems in place to detect potential harm events before harm reaches our patients or employees?
- Does our organization practice mindfulness and follow the HRO principles?

Additionally, the voice of the customer should also be a guiding light for HROs. The idea of "what matters most to our patients and their families" was best captured by Brilli et al. [11] and then later reemphasized in an IHI white paper [12] (Fig. 15.3): "Keep me safe, help me navigate my care, help keep me well, treat me with respect, and provide me with the right care." This model, unlike the previous STEEEP (safe-timely-effective-efficient-equitable-patient centered) terminology, better captures patient expectations with regard to growth, evolution, and complexity of healthcare delivery. Therefore, all improvement projects need to fall under one or several of these five aforementioned patient and community-centric categories. Board members need to ask whether clinical and nonclinical projects are aligned with these perspectives. Workforce or employee safety, while not directly mentioned in this model, can be included under the "keep me safe" and "treat me with respect" domains.

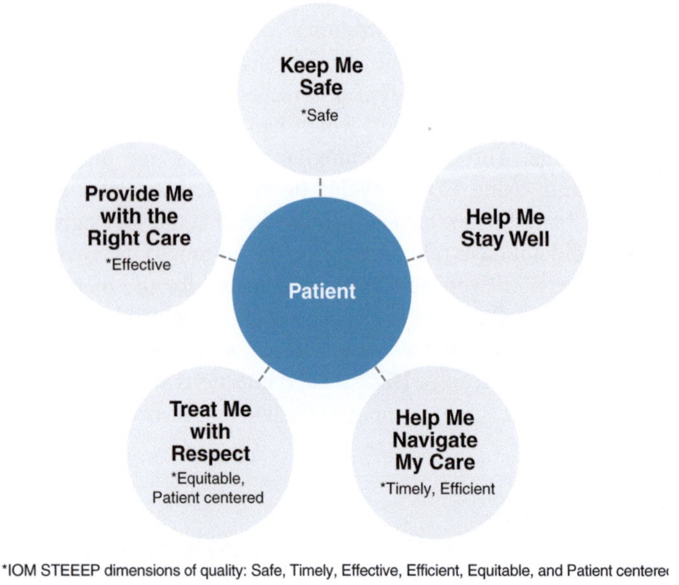

Fig. 15.3 Core components of quality from the patient's perspective. (Source: Daley Ullem et al. [12]. (Available on ihi.org). This figure is used with permission from the Institute for Healthcare Improvement)

Society has tasked healthcare systems to become "learning systems," where structures, processes, and outcomes are optimized and constantly reviewed, to support an organizational cadence of continuous process improvement [9, 13–15]. No adverse event should ever recur if the root cause is uncovered through structured problem-solving, and inefficient or unsafe processes are improved. This is a win for the patient, the providers, and all other stakeholders!

An organization can only deliver results it has been designed to deliver. This concept has been enshrined by many prominent leaders. Dr. Avedis Donabedian best described this relationship between structure, process, and outcomes [16]. Good structures enable good processes which, in turn, give good results. In other words, if an organization is not getting the results it wants, it cannot just continue to push its frontline people to work harder. The problem, more often than not, lies in the preexisting organizational structures and processes, not with the workers. Deming highlighted this point in *The New Economics* [2]. He also consistently maintained that the majority of an organization's problems are due to the processes that management puts in place and not the people. In *The New Economics* he also writes, "Ninety-five percent of changes made by management today make no improvement."

The Baldrige Performance Excellence Program (BPEP), in Gaithersburg, MD, provides another useful framework for performance excellence. The Baldrige criteria were the outgrowth of a national program sponsored by former President Ronald Reagan [17]. This program and its framework have endured the test of time, undergone multiple revisions to keep it current, and also trained many examiners to these standards. The program teaches its applicants and examiners to assess organizational processes using the ADLI mnemonic, which stands for **A**pproach-**D**eployment-**L**earning-**I**ntegration.

Under **A**pproach, BPEP asks organizations:

- How do you accomplish the organization's work?
- How systematic and effective are your approaches?

Similarly, under **D**eployment BPEP asks:

- How consistently are your key approaches used in relevant parts of your organization?

With **L**earning, it asks:

- How well have you evaluated and improved your key approaches?
- How well has improvement been shared within your organization?
- How has knowledge led to innovation?

The **I**ntegration aspect of BPEP asks:

- How do your approaches reflect your current and future organizational needs?
- How well are processes and operations harmonized across your organization to achieve key organization-wide goals?

Organizational processes that meet all the key components of ADLI are considered to be effective and systematic. They undergo continuous improvement as organizational learning occurs from safety events, daily operations, and customer feedback. The resulting innovative ideas are shared and deployed throughout the organization. These processes are standardized and repeated with minimal variation.

An organization's results reflect its overall structure and processes, as described in the Donabedian principles mentioned earlier. An organization cannot expect good results without attention and investment in its structure and processes. Lloyd [18] added a third component to Donabedian's model by adding culture (C) to the equation (S + P + C = O). Without an explicit focus on the cultures, both formal and informal, an organization's structures and processes will not function in an optimal manner.

While the Baldrige ADLI is the mnemonic used to assess processes, *LeTCI* is the mnemonic used to assess the results of an organization and stands for **Le**vels-**T**rends-**C**omparisons-**I**ntegration. LeTCI is often stated as "Let's See," which reflects its use in the review of results. **L**evels pertain to the current organizational performance using an understandable and accepted measurement scale. **T**rends refer to the rate of improvement, or sustainment, of good outcomes. **C**omparisons ask that results are presented along with other relative reference data. **I**ntegration refers to the magnitude with which results address and align to improve system performance goals relating to patients, team members, and other stakeholders. Results cannot be properly interpreted unless the ADLI components are provided.

Points to Ponder

- Which core components of quality from a patient's perspective pertain to the project in question?
- When processes are discussed, use ADLI to critically evaluate them.
- When results or outcomes are presented, use LeTCI to critically evaluate them.

Science of Improvement

The *science of improvement* (SOI) provides an overarching discipline for organizing all of the frameworks referenced above. The history of the SOI is rich in both theory and application [19] and depends upon two crucial components. First, engage subject matter experts, with their experience and knowledge, to develop and guide successful change resulting in improvement. Second, ensure that the adjustments will result in effective change by utilizing Dr. W. Edwards Deming's "System of Profound Knowledge" (SOPK) (Fig. 15.4). SOPK is comprised of four key components: (1) appreciation of a system, (2) understanding variation, (3) theory of knowledge, and (4) human behavior (originally called psychology by Deming). Expertise with the SOPK, combined with sub-

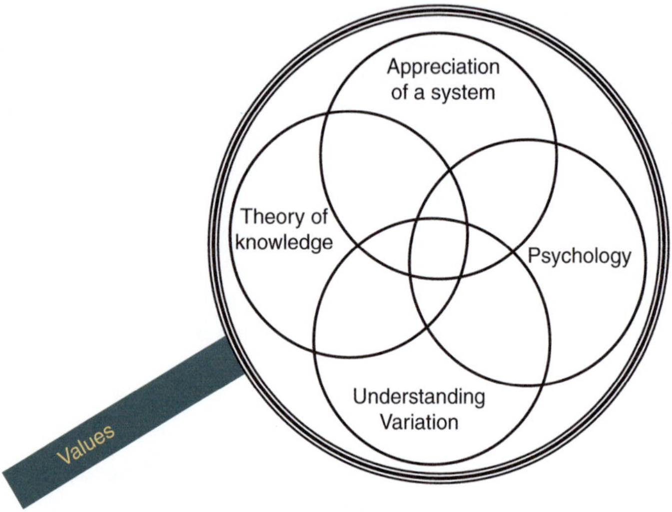

Fig. 15.4 Deming's System of Profound Knowledge. (From Langley et al. [5] – printed with permission from John Wiley & Sons, Inc.)

ject matter expertise, facilitates creative thinking, innovation, and improvement [5].

Appreciation of a System The appreciation of a system encourages recognition of processes involving flow, demand, supply, and decision-making. A central principle of the SOI is that every system is perfectly designed to deliver the results it produces. Donabedian principles are also part of the appreciation of a system. If the outcomes of the system are suboptimal, then the system usually needs to be changed to better optimize its results. Additionally, there may be unexpected consequences upstream, or downstream, from a changed process for which one must be prepared [5, 16].

Understanding the Variation Variation exists! Everything we do in medicine has variation. For instance, every time we sign a document by hand, there is some minor variation in that signature from the previous time it was used. Two clinicians doing the same procedure will have some variation between them, or each time they perform the procedure independently vs. with a colleague. Improvement focuses on reducing variation in processes. Figure 15.5 provides run charts, showing the variation of two units with regard to their productivity (run charts will be explained in greater detail later in the chapter). In which unit (A or B) would it be easier to achieve the target of 70%? In Unit A (Fig. 15.5a), for example, there is considerable variation in the process represented with extreme high and low points, which make this process more difficult to improve. On the other hand, unit B (Fig. 15.5b) exhibits less variation, making improvement potentially easier to achieve.

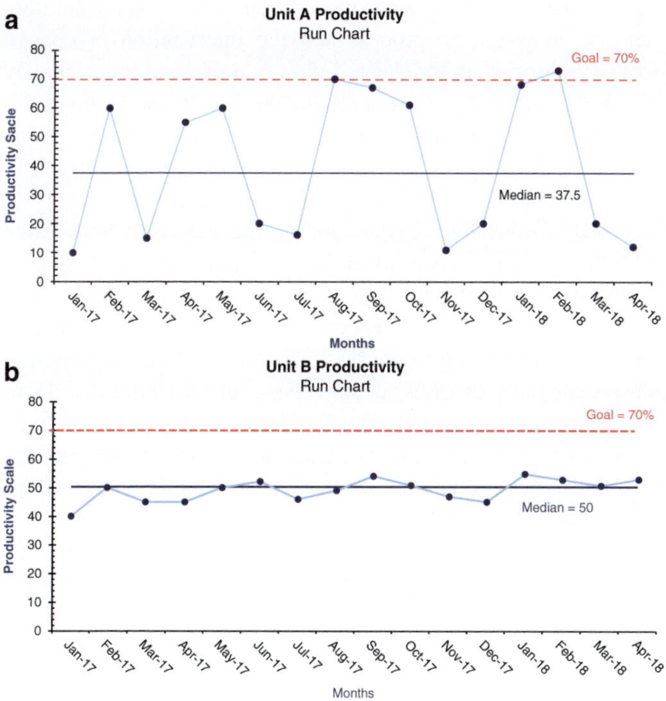

Fig. 15.5 (**a** and **b**) Reducing variation and moving to a new level of performance

Understanding the types of variation is crucial. There are usually two patterns in data variation, those that are predictable and those that are unpredictable. Similarly, there are two causes for these types of variation: common cause and special cause. These statistical concepts were detailed by Dr. Walter Shewhart in his classic book *Economic Control of Quality of Manufactured Product* [20]. Common cause variation is predictable and inherent to the process or system and, therefore, affects all components of the process and resulting outcomes. Special cause variation, on the other hand, produces results that are unstable and unpredictable. Special cause variation may be unexpected (e.g., a train wreck that causes many patients to be sent to your emergency room), and not part of the normal functioning of a process or system. Special cause variation can also occur when you deliberately intervene to change a process and the intervention or change moves the process in the desired direction of goodness. The key point is that variation exists in all that we do. Understanding variation requires, therefore, looking at data over time not in the aggregate. More will be said about this critical point shortly.

Theory of Knowledge Understanding the theory of knowledge and how team members think and learn are crucial to driving successful improvement. Many people assume that this component is not practical because it references "theory." This conclusion is far from what Dr. Deming meant by this component. It is very practical. We all have theories, perspectives, and assumptions about how work gets done or not done. Our "view of the world," as some sociologists call it, provides the lens through which we view the work and how it functions. Doctors have theories about nurses. Nurses have theories about doctors. Both have theories about management. Whose theory is "the right one?" Theories about the world provide a foundation for learning and change. As Dr. George Box, a famous statistician, once said, "All models are wrong, but some are useful." [21] We need to explore the theories that we all have about how work gets done or not done. Additionally, the more knowledge that is gained about a particular system and its processes, the better the likelihood that any proposed change will result in the desired improvement.

Human Behavior Initially in Dr. Deming's early writings (e.g., see *The New Economics*, 1994 [2]), he referred to this component as psychology. He later revised the name of this component to be human behavior to reflect a broader and more encompassing concept to include culture, motivation, joy in work, and the destructive forces of management. Understanding human behavior and organizational culture will permit the creation of proper strategies to motivate stakeholders and team members around an improvement focus. Casual analyses of harm events have shown the importance of organizational culture in achieving strategic goals. Culture has many definitions but is best described as the way people behave when no one is looking. Building a culture of mutual accountability requires trust and respect among all stakeholders. Board members need to keep culture in the forefront and help build bridges to facilitate improvement and positive change. They also need to realize the popular statement that "culture eats strategy for lunch!"

An understanding of the four components of the SOPK, and their respective interactions through structured learning, can prepare an improvement team for any potential hurdles they may face. As a board member, it is important to understand that system improvement requires local subject matter experts and the SOPK, resulting in greater self-learning, system understanding and capability to drive improvement. An essential aspect of using the SOPK is appreciating the interaction of the four components. Being an expert in one or even two of the components will not lead to organizational success.

Points to Ponder

- How are the various components of the System of Profound Knowledge incorporated into a project plan? Specifically, describe the system that is the focus of the change initiative, including its processes, outcomes, customers, and stakeholders.
- Are there set standards from which you are measuring variation and driving improvement?
- What types of variation are present? Common cause or special cause?

- How will improvement and learning be facilitated?
- What is the culture in the area where the project is occurring? Will the local team members be supportive of the improvement efforts?

Constancy of Purpose

The various well-known approaches, or models, used to drive quality strategies and initiatives all have utility and have been used successfully by organizations to achieve the stages in Deming's chain reaction (Fig. 15.1). However, organizations need a single preferred organizational improvement model to standardize their messages and methods of improvement and to ensure that everyone is speaking the same "language." A single preferred model leads to what Dr. Deming called "constancy of purpose" [1, 2]. There are several well-known improvement models or approaches currently in use that were mentioned previously. In this chapter, we are focusing on the details of one of the most widely used approaches, the Model for Improvement (MFI) shown in Fig. 15.6.

Created by the Associates for Process Improvement (API) [5] and widely adapted for use by the Institute for Healthcare Improvement (IHI), this model has been successfully used by many health and social service organizations around the world to improve. The MFI has two major components. The first component consists of three questions that serve as a road map for guiding the organization's quality journey. The three questions are:

1. What are we trying to accomplish? This is the aim of this improvement work.
2. How will we know that a change is an improvement? This is the measurement question.
3. What changes can we make that will result in improvement? This is the action.

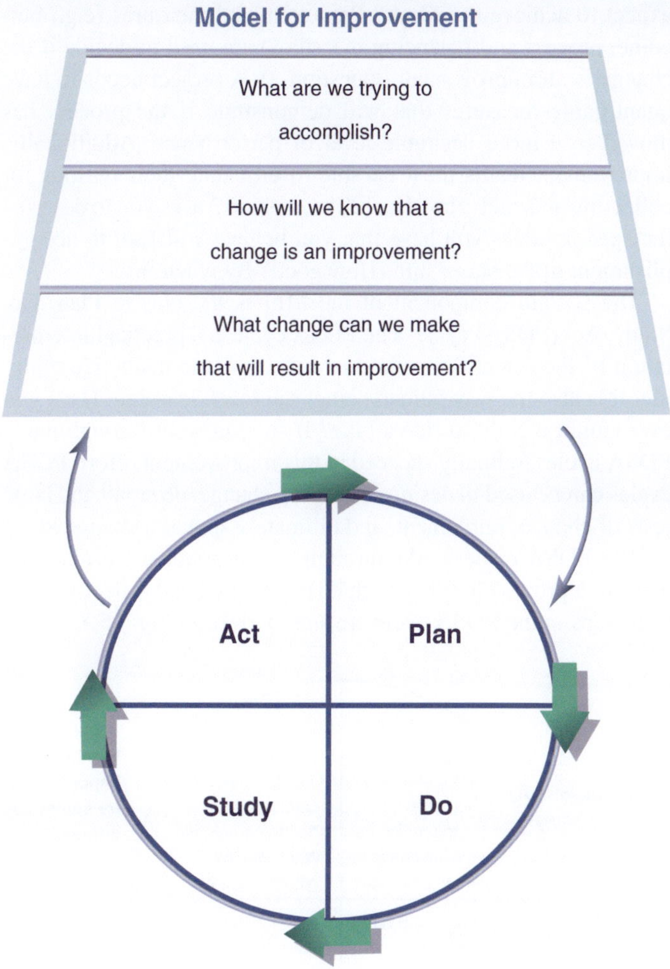

Fig. 15.6 IHI/API Model for Improvement. (From Langley et al. [5] – printed with permission from John Wiley & Sons, Inc.)

A useful aim statement (Question 1) is usually based on being **s**pecific, **m**easurable, **a**chievable, **r**ealistic, and **t**imely (i.e., SMART). Two key questions related to an aim statement are the following: (1) How good do you want to be? (2) By when do you expect to achieve the result? Predetermined measures (e.g., outcome, process and balancing measures) are used to decide if the change is an improvement (Question 2). A project needs to have quantifiable measures that will demonstrate if the process has moved to a more desirable level of performance. Additionally, improvement teams must be able to articulate their reasons for collecting and analyzing data [22]. Question 3 asks you to describe the specific ideas you have that you believe will lead to accomplishment of the stated aim (How good? By when?).

The second component of the MFI is the classic Plan, Do, Study, Act (PDSA) cycle. The PDSA cycle is a practical interpretation of the scientific method of inductive and deductive thinking. It is also the way human beings approach learning. Have you ever taught a child to ride a bike? If so, you went through many PDSA cycles to finally succeed in this improvement effort. PDSA cycles can be used to design or develop change, do small and large tests of change, implement, and ultimately spread a change idea.

The PDSA cycle works through action-oriented learning and leads to a process for change that is structured and reflective. The four steps in the PDSA cycle are summarized in Fig. 15.7.

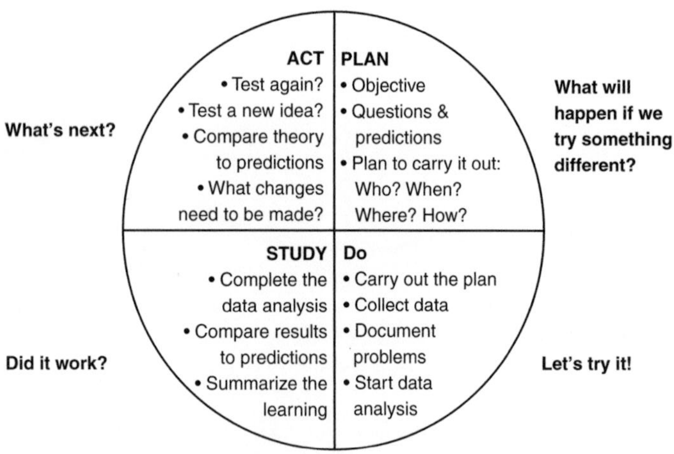

Fig. 15.7 The components of the PDSA cycle. (Used with permission of Robert Lloyd, PhD and Jones & Bartlett Learning. Source: Lloyd [3], 342. Reprinted with permission, www.jblearning.com)

The PDSA cycle is not a one-time event. It is an iterative cycle designed to help teams minimize the risk and consequences of failures. Through multiple iterations of the PDSA Cycle, a team discovers what works and does not work (a failed test). By refining the change idea and increasing the size and scope of subsequent test cycles, a stronger degree of belief is obtained by the team that the improvement idea works not only in the pilot area but also in other areas that have different operating conditions. Once the change idea has been tested under different conditions (e.g., day, afternoon, and night shifts; weekdays vs. weekends; or with different patient populations), it is time to consider implementing the new idea and determining if the gains initially observed can be maintained. If so, then it is time to consider spreading the new idea to other units, clinics, or facilities. This sequence of improvement can be viewed as a series of steps as shown in Fig. 15.8. Note that as you move from initial testing on

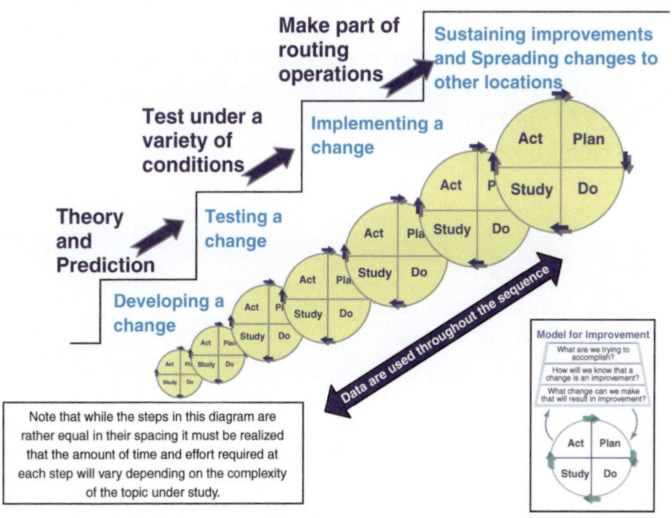

Fig. 15.8 The sequence of improvement. (Developed by Dr. R. Lloyd for workshop presentation on quality improvement measurement at the Royal Free NHS Foundation Trust, London, June 20–23, 2018. Used with permission from Dr. Lloyd)

a small scale to testing under different conditions, then to implementation, and finally to spreading a new idea, the PDSA cycles become larger and more involved. This journey also requires the use of data throughout in order to learn if the change idea has made a difference. It is not a difficult journey but one that requires the integration of testing theories, making predictions, and using data to determine if a change has made a difference in performance.

Many organizations have chosen to create their own improvement methodologies based on the PDSA cycle. The Children's Hospital of the King's Daughters Health System, for example, uses an improvement methodology shown in Fig. 15.9, which combines the Model for Improvement, Toyota Production System, and Lean Six Sigma.

All improvement methods help drive change through structured problem-solving during which a complex problem is broken down into small manageable parts. Each is then addressed with the understanding that small changes, when taken as a whole, lead to breakthrough transformation and innovation. As mentioned previously, the PDSA cycle is the vehicle by which ideas created during the three questions of the Model for Improvement (Fig. 15.6) are tested and further learning results. Each PDSA cycle builds upon the next.

Points to Ponder

- What is the organization's preferred standard methodology for improvement?
- Ask all three questions from the Model for Improvement (Fig. 15.6).
- Who will go out and collect the data?
- Do you already know the baseline data?
- How will the data be used to make a difference?
- Are there stakeholders participating from all of the areas that will be impacted by your improvement project?

Plan / Do / Study / Act	1 Identify the Opportunity	2 Understand the Process	3 Establish the Plan	4 PDSA Cycles	5 Sustain Improvement
	PLAN	PLAN	PLAN	DO & STUDY	ACT
	MODEL FOR IMPROVEMENT Question #1: What are we trying to accomplish? *AIM statement*	MODEL FOR IMPROVEMENT Question #2: How do we know a change is an improvement? *Select measures*	MODEL FOR IMPROVEMENT Question #3: What changes will result in a measurable improvement? *Select changes*	Question #4: How do we do and study our proposed chages?	Question #5: Implement, Sustain and Spreading Improvement
Key Points	• Identity opportunity for improvement • Ensure strategic alignment with oranizational goals • Examine causal analyses and regulatory requirements	• Develop a picture of the current state of the process	• Develop a picture of the future state of the process • Identify a way to measure the defects/opportunities for improvement (OFIs) of the process • Identify gaps for measurable improvement	• Test changes • Test under different conditions • Monitor performance	• Implement • Monitor performance
Methods	• Voice of Customer Techniques (Patient, Family, and Frontline Team Members) • Brainstorming • Stakeholderr Analysis • Team Formation • Prioritization Matrix	• SIPOC (Supplier-Inputs-Process-Outputs-Customers) • Flow Diagram Forms for collecting data • Process Maps • Observations – Gemba • Cause and Effect Diagrams • Pareto Chart • Run and Control Charts	• Project Charter • SMART Aim Statement • Key Driver Diagram • Problem Solving • Gantt Chart	• PDSA Forms • PDSA Ramps • Run and Control Charts	• ACT: Adopt, Adapt or Abandon • Discuss spread opportunities • Standardize processes through Job Instruction • Policy Evaluation • Celebrate success • Debrief QI team

Fig. 15.9 CHKD improvement methodology. (Courtesy of the Department of Quality and Safety, Children's Hospital of The King's Daughters, Norfolk, VA)

The Board's Critical Role in Analyzing Data Over Time

Every board meeting should have time on the agenda dedicated to reviewing data. During this period, the members are asked to make decisions based upon what the data reveals. Are we on target? Have we met the strategic goals? Are we better now than we were last board meeting? How would you know? Unfortunately, if you are presented with aggregated data and summary statistics comparing this quarter with the previous quarter, you will never know the answers to these questions.

Data presented in tabular formats or with aggregated summary statistics will never help you determine if you are delivering excellence to those you serve or the impact of process improvement efforts. Aggregated data and summary statistics can only lead to judgement, not to improvement. Yet many organizations are wedded to using the mean, median, mode, minimum, maximum, range, or standard deviation in board reports to make decisions about the variation in their data. Some even go so far as to use tests of significance (e.g., *p*-values) to "prove" that there is a difference between the last quarter's figures and the current quarter's results. Dr. Deming was very clear about this point. He wrote [1]:

> Students are not warned in classes nor in the books that for analytic purposes, distributions and calculations of mean, mode, standard deviation, chi-square, t-test, etc. serve no useful purpose for improvement of a process unless the data were produced in a state of statistical control. Aggregated data, therefore, can only lead to judgment not to improvement. (1992: 312)

The most popular approach to presenting aggregated data in healthcare board and management meetings, however, is not with summary statistics but rather with ever popular red/yellow/green format. Figure 15.10 presents a typical red/yellow/green display of data. Charts that follow this familiar format do not allow board members to make informed decisions about the variation that produced the results. All that can be concluded is that a particular

Organization Dashboard Summary
Quarterly Performance Against Plan

GOALS	Organization Total				FY	Annual Budget/	
	Q1	Q2	Q3	Q4	TOTAL	Goal	Variance
FINANCIAL							
Net Gain	25,000	30,000	30,000	28,000	113,000	113,000	1%
VOLUME & PRODUCTIVITY							
ADV	275	275	285	300	285	300	-5%
Deliveries	200	200	225	250	875	1,000	-13%
Provider Productivity	4,000	3,900	4,000	4,100	4,000	4,000	0%
Days to 3rd - 1 slot	15	13	14	15	14	15.0	-5%
Days to 3rd - 2 slot	25	23	21	20	22	20.0	11%
% No Show/Cancel	28%	26%	26%	25%	26%	25%	5%
% Same Day/Next Day/Triage	10%	13%	18%	17%	15%	15%	-3%
PATIENT SATISFACTION							
Survey Response	750	750	1,000	1,000	3,500	4,000	-13%
Overall Rating	4.6	4.6	4.5	4.6	4.6	4.7	-3%
Would Recommend	4.7	4.7	4.6	4.6	4.7	4.7	-1%
EMPLOYEE SATISFACTION	3.9		4.0	4.0	4.0	4.0	-1%
CLINICAL HEALTH OUTCOMES							
Core Indicators	50	50	50	50	50		
Core Indicators Goal Achieved	40	38	37	36	38		
% Core Indicators Goal Achieved	80%	76%	74%	72%	76%	80%	-6%
Priority Indicators Goal Achieved	19	19	18	17	18		
% Priority Indicators Goal Achieved	95%	95%	90%	85%	91%	95%	-4%

Key:

(green)	Goal Achieved
(yellow)	Goal within 5% of Achieved
(red)	Goal NOT Achieved (beyond 5%)

Fig. 15.10 A typical red/yellow/green graphic of performance. (Developed for this chapter and used with permission of Robert Lloyd, PhD)

measure is above, near, or below a target. Nothing is learned about the inherent variation in the process that produced the resultant red/yellow/green rankings. There are three major problems with using this format to display aggregated data:

1. Data are usually shown in aggregations that are lagged and that compare data by large blocks of time (e.g., this year compared to last year, this month compared to the same month a year ago or this quarter compared to the last quarter).
2. The inherent variation in the data is suppressed in a red/yellow/green format. If improvement is the objective, then the variation that produced the observed results must be made visible and understood.
3. Arbitrary cut points are usually established to determine when a measure is classified as being in the red, yellow, or green categories. An interesting aspect of making the cut points is that a majority of the time the targets or goals that determine the cut points are established around whole numbers divisible by 5 (e.g., 85%, 90%, 95%) which makes no sense. Targets and goals should be established based on the inherent variation that exists in the current process and the capability of this process to achieve the stated target or goal. Targets and goals are too often removed from the current capability of a process to achieve the desired target or goal. Thus, many targets and goals can be classified as being "arbitrary and capricious." With respect to goals Deming wrote:

   > Goals are necessary for you and for me, but numerical goals set for other people, without a road map to reach the goal, have effects opposite to the effects sought. (1992: 69)

Therefore, the key questions board members should be asking when presented with aggregated data and summary statistical or red/yellow/green graphics are:

- By what method do you plan to achieve better performance?
- Given the variation that produced this result, is the current process capable of ever achieving the target or goal?

If the board and senior management are genuinely committed to making quality the organization's central business strategy, then they need to move away from static displays of data with summary statistics and view the organization's performance in a dynamic manner. This comes by presenting data on statistical process control (SPC) charts, which show the variation that lives in the data and enables leaders to make more informed decisions about the probability of achieving performance targets and goals. These decisions cannot be enabled when data are presented in aggregated formats with summary statistics or red/yellow/green graphics.

The history of analyzing data in a dynamic rather than static fashion traces its roots back to the early 1920s when Dr. Walter Shewhart proposed to the management of Western Electric, later to become Bell Laboratories and then AT&T, the fundamentals of what we know today as modern industrial quality control [20, 23]. Shewhart posed a very simple question to the leaders of Western Electric, "What is the variation in one system over time?" With this simple question, he was able to inspire Western Electric's management team to learn about the variation inherent in their systems rather than reporting the total number of defective products produced each quarter or month.

A variety of analytic methods are part of what has become known as SPC methods and tools. Principal among SPC tools are run charts and Shewhart (control) charts. Figure 15.11 summarizes the basic elements of each form of charting.

A run chart has several important components, as described in the top portion of Fig. 15.11. When an organization is ready to apply control, classically known as Shewhart, charts to its measures, however, deeper knowledge of SPC is required, because there are many control charts to choose from. The most appropriate chart selection depends on the type of measure being analyzed (e.g., a count, a percent, a rate, an index or score, or the time between defects or errors). The technical details behind run and control charts are described in very practical terms for healthcare professionals in *Quality Health Care: A Guide to Developing and Using Indicators* [3] and *The Health Care Data Guide: Learning from Data for Improvement* [6].

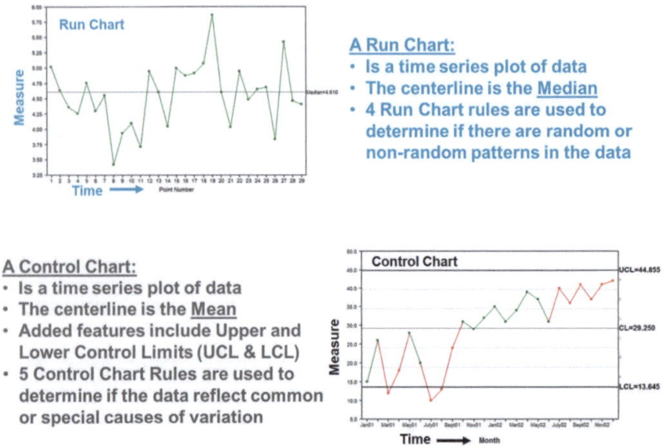

Fig. 15.11 Primary statistical tools used to analyze quality. (Developed by Dr. R. Lloyd for workshop presentation on quality improvement measurement at the Royal Free NHS Foundation Trust, London, June 20–23, 2018. Used with permission from Dr. Lloyd)

Most board members do not need, or even want, to know the technical details behind run chart and Shewhart construction. If the organization is truly committed to quality as its business strategy, there will be medical leaders or individuals in the quality or performance improvement departments who have studied the proper use and application of the charts and know how to understand variation statistically. What board members need to know, however, is how to interpret and learn from the charts when they are presented. This is achieved by understanding variation conceptually and being able to recognize the differences between common cause and special cause variation.

Understanding Variation Conceptually

Variation exists in all that we do even in the simplest of activities. For example, consider writing your name. This is a simple activity that you probably do each day. Imagine that your annual performance review, however, was based on being able to write the first letter of your first name three times with no variation in the form, structure, or overall appearance of the letter. If you are able to perform this simple task, you will receive a 50% increase in your salary. Remember that there can be no variation in the letters. Give it a try. But wait, there is a second part to your performance evaluation. Place your pen or pencil in your opposite hand and write the same letter three times. To receive the 50% increase in salary, all six letters must be *exactly* the same with no variation. How many of you passed the performance evaluation test? Even the letters written with your dominant hand are not identical and show variation.

Dr. Walter Shewhart proposed a way to think about variation back in the early 1920s.

Shewhart's recommendation for creating efficient and effective processes was very simple. He maintained that if you understand the variation that occurs within a process or system, you will be able to make appropriate management decisions that will produce high-quality products and services. Shewhart distinguished two types of variation, assignable and unassignable. These terms were later revised by Deming to the more popular terms used today, common and special causes of variation [2, 20, 24]. Figure 15.12 provides a summary of the characteristics associated with common and special causes of variation.

Common Cause Variation

- Is inherent in the design of the process
- Is due to regular, natural or ordinary causes
- Affects all the outcomes of a process
- Results in a "stable" process that is predictable
- Also known as random or unassignable variation

Special Cause Variation

- Is due to irregular or unnatural causes that are not in inherent in the design of the process
- Affect some, but not necessarily all aspects of the process
- Results in an "unstable" process that is not predictable
- Also known as non-random or assignable variation

Fig. 15.12 Types of variation. (Developed by Dr. R. Lloyd for workshop presentation on quality improvement measurement at the Royal Free NHS Foundation Trust, London, June 20–23, 2018. Used with permission from Dr. Lloyd)

According to Lloyd [3], it is possible to make predictions, within statistical limits, about a process that has only common cause variation. In a common cause system, there are no indications of special cause, because the variation results only from chance fluctuation in the data. Your morning commute to work provides an excellent practical example of understanding variation. If you ask people, "How long does it take you to get to work in the morning?" most respond, "Oh about (fill in the blank) minutes." Each day's commute is not exactly the same number of minutes. One day it takes a little longer to get to work and then the next day a little less time. There is fluctuation from day to day, but your commute times exhibit a random (common cause) pattern that centers about an average commute time. Then, there is the day when you encounter a bad accident on the highway you typically travel. Traffic is not moving and you keep looking at your watch wondering if you will get to work in time to lead your team meeting. The accident represents an irregular event, which results in an unpredictable commute time. You are now experiencing a special cause in your morning commute.

The key thing to remember about understanding variation, however, is that common cause variation does not mean that the performance of the process is good or even acceptable. It only means only that the process is stable and, therefore, predictable. A process can be predictably bad. For example, a patient may have blood pressure readings that are stable and very predictable but at an unacceptably high level (e.g., a systolic pressure that averages 175 with a minimum at 165 and a maximum at 185). It is stable and therefore predictable but unacceptable clinically. The same could be true for cholesterol, white blood cell counts, or blood glucose levels. In all these cases, we would need to shift the various process outputs to more acceptable levels of performance. This is what quality improvement is designed to do. Remember, though, common cause means stable and predictable, not necessarily acceptable [3].

Making the Appropriate Response

Leaders should respond appropriately to the variation that lives in their data. Table 15.1 summarizes the response options when confronted with common cause and special cause variation. The right choice when common cause variation is observed is to either continue to monitor the process (if the performance is acceptable) or redesign the process (if the performance is unacceptable). The appropriate response to when special cause variation is detected is to investigate the reasons why the special cause(s) occurred. Since special cause variation makes a process unstable and unpredictable, attempts to improve the process will only lead to wasted time, effort, and money, as well as an increase in variation. The responsibility of the board, therefore, is to make appropriate decisions when shown performance data. Statistical thinking and knowledge of common and special cause variation will serve as a reliable road map for making sound decisions.

Table 15.1 Appropriate responses to common and special causes of variation

	Is the proces stable?	
	YES	NO
Type of variation	Common Cause	Special Cause
Right Choice	Monitor or change the process	Investigate the origin of the special cause variation
Wrong Choice	Treat common cause variation as if it were special (tampering)	Change the process
Consequences of making the wrong choice	*Increased variation!*	*Wasted resources!* *(time, effort, resources morale)*

Used with permission of Robert Lloyd, PhD and Jones & Bartlett Learning: Source: Lloyd [3], 182. Reprinted with permission, www.jblearning.com

Application of Statistical Thinking

Returning to the initial example of patient falls mentioned earlier, a run chart was created to represent the data (Fig. 15.13). When the number of falls was increasing, we see an increasing trend in the data (i.e., ≥5 consecutive increasing points, the first circled region (gray) on chart), which shows the time when the new cleaner was implemented and the resulting increase in patient falls. The second circled region (green) of the chart shows that there was also an upward shift in the number of falls (i.e., ≥6 consecutive points above the median). Then, the third circled region (green) shows that when the facility went back to using the old floor cleaner, the number of falls shifted downward (i.e., ≥6 consecutive points below the median).

Next, an examination of patient falls data, discussed throughout this chapter and displayed as a Shewhart control chart in Fig. 15.14, displays two regions (circled with dashed lines) that resemble special cause variation. As discussed earlier in the chapter, a decision was made to change the floor cleaner, which resulted in the increase in falls and a special cause variation (≥6 consecutive increasing data points), as represented by the three data points outside the UCL. The decision to revert to the original cleaner occurred after the RCA was undertaken. This latter change

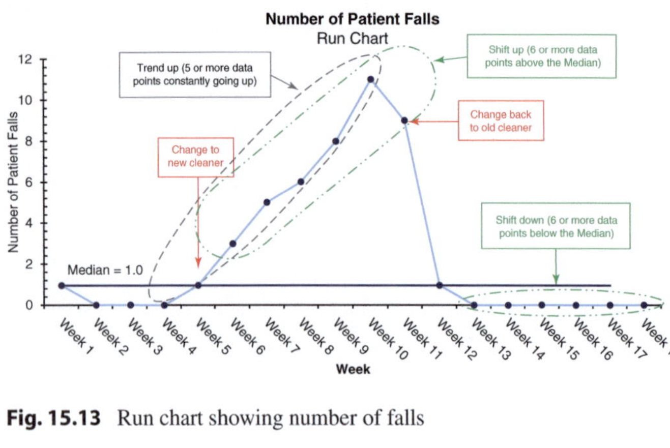

Fig. 15.13 Run chart showing number of falls

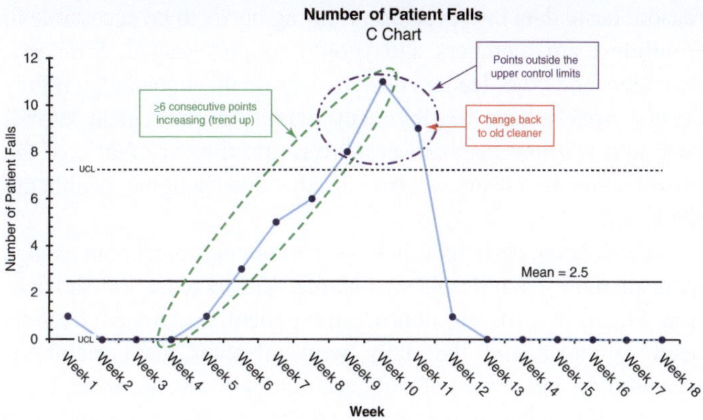

Fig. 15.14 Shewhart control chart of the number of patient falls

then resulted in a decline in the number of falls and another area of a special cause, as represented by the six points below the centerline (i.e., a downward shift in the data). As mentioned earlier, a special cause can be good or bad.

Note that the data used in this patient falls example and mentioned throughout this chapter was intentionally kept simple. In reality, however, the data may show considerable variation after a single intervention, necessitating further problem-solving and additional interventions to arrive at a desired outcome. We hope that this example encourages the reader to seek additional knowledge about the application of statistical process control methods to performance indicators.

Building a Learning Organization

Peter Senge in *The Fifth Discipline: The Art & Practice of The Learning Organization* [13] is well known for challenging management to build "learning organizations," but as he writes, many organizations suffer from what he calls "learning disabilities." The proper analysis and display of data are needed to optimally drive improvement and become a learning organization. After all, you cannot improve what you cannot see or understand. For this reason, basic data interpretation training needs to be accessible to frontline team members and should be encouraged. Similarly, managers and other leaders need to acquire this knowledge if they do not already have it. Obviously, quality improvement knowledge and learning needs to be woven into the very fabric of the organization to ensure success in the everchanging healthcare landscape.

Additionally, participation in improvement projects can engage team members, build cohesive teams, and increase job satisfaction which, in turn, can improve the patient experience. Leaders need to understand the daily work of their team members. Recognition and reward of daily accomplishments is crucial. Let's face it – complaints and negative results are often communicated with greater frequency than positive comments to frontline staff. Daily organizational safety briefs, for example, can serve to share safety stories as well as highlight the great work and good safety catches that likely occur at all organizations but are underreported. Kouzes and Posner, in *The Leadership Challenge* [25], discussed the value of leaders in encouraging team members.

The participation of the hospital board in the celebration of success can also be invaluable. Celebrations can be simple or elaborate [26, 27]. Team members appreciate the presence and participation of the board in recognition events. Simple congratulatory notes from board members are also memorable and cherished. Board members can participate in hospital leadership rounds, during which they can start dialogues and ask questions which promote team building and positive organizational culture. From such experiences, board members may gather stories of challenges that were overcome with resulting success. These narratives can then be shared at various venues, especially with other health systems and at community meetings.

The journey to becoming a high-reliability organization is fraught with many challenges. Recognition of success by board members can help build a joyful and engaged workforce. This, in turn, fosters team member engagement with patient experience, organizational strategic goals, fellow team members, and further goal setting. For this reason, everyone involved with the organizations' journey wins, regardless of their role and position within the organization. Life and joy in work need to be celebrated!

In conclusion, a hospital board can drive innovation, safety, and quality just by asking thoughtful questions. Board members do not need to be masters of quality improvement and safety principles, as that is the role of the local quality and safety leaders. However, inquisitive questions, especially about the variation inherent in the organization's data, can promote further discussion and system learning, resolve issues, lead to innovation and better communication, and create opportunities for growth and improvement. Questions, especially from board members, demonstrate engagement, and the ensuing dialogue can be a positive boost for an organization's culture and journey toward becoming a high-reliability organization.

Dr. W. Edwards Deming once said, "*A bad system will beat a good person every time*" [28]. Hence, hospital boards need to engage their frontline teams and leaders and create collaborative learning systems that are focused on continuous improvement. We know that our patients, their families, and our communities expect this. Dr. Deming encouraged a questioning attitude – "*If you do not know how to ask the right question, you discover nothing*" [28]. So, next time you sit in a board meeting during a presentation, especially one focused on quality, safety, or patient and staff feedback data, remember the positive ramifications of asking questions about common and special cause variation.

Points to Ponder

- Is data interpretation training available to leadership and frontline team members?
- In the run chart, did you find any nonrandom points in your data assessment? Do you have an explanation for them?
- In your statistical process control (SPC) chart, do you have an explanation for any special cause variation?
- Based on your analyses, what are the next steps and why?
- How are we going to celebrate those good results?

Acknowledgments The authors would like to acknowledge Adam Campbell, Kate Conrad, Regina Dawson, Tamara Johnson, Christopher Mangum, Karen Mitchell, Jeanann Pardue, Lisa Parker, Elizabeth Pittman, and Teresa Saulnier for their careful reading and feedback on this chapter when it was in development.

References

1. Deming WE. Out of the crisis. 1st ed. Cambridge, MA: MIT Press; 1992.
2. Deming WE. The New Economics. 2nd ed. Cambridge, MA: MIT Press; 1994.
3. Lloyd RC. Quality health care: a guide to developing and using indicators. Burlington, MA: Jones and Bartlett Learning; 2019.
4. Associates in Process Improvement. Quality as a business strategy: an overview. 2017: API, 115 East Fifth Street, Suite 300, Austin, Texas 78701. (http://apiweb.org/index.php/resources/publications).
5. Langley GJ, Moen RD, Nolan KM, Nolan TW, Norman CL, Provost LP. The improvement guide: a practical approach to enhancing organizational performance. 2nd ed. San Francisco: Jossey-Bass; 2009.
6. Provost LP, Murray SK. The health care data guide: learning from data for improvement. San Francisco, CA: Jossey Bass; 2011.
7. Kohn LT, Corrigan JM, Donaldson MS. To err is human: building a safer health system. Washington, DC: National Academies Press; 2000.
8. Millar R, Mannion R, Freeman T, Davies HT. Hospital board oversight of quality and patient safety: a narrative review and synthesis of recent empirical research. Milbank Q. 2013;91(4):738–70.
9. Committee on Quality of Health Care in America. Crossing the quality chasm: a new health system for the 21st century. Washington, DC: The National Academies Press; 2001.
10. Weick KE, Sutcliffe KM. Managing the unexpected: resilient performance in an age of uncertainty. San Francisco: Wiley; 2007.
11. Brilli RJ, Allen S, Davis JT. Revisiting the quality chasm. Pediatrics. 2014;133(5):763–5.
12. Daley Ullem E, Gandhi TK, Mate K, Whittington J, Renton M, Huebner J. Framework for effective board governance of health system quality. In: IHI white paper. Boston, MA: Institute for Healthcare Improvement; 2018. p. 1–36.
13. Senge PM. The fifth discipline: the art and practice of the learning organization. New York: Crown Business Publishing; 2006.
14. Scholtes PR. The team handbook: how to use teams to improve quality. Methuen, MA: Goal/QPC; 1988.
15. Covey SR. The 7 habits of highly effective people: powerful lessons in personal change. New York: Simon and Schuster; 2013.

16. Ayanian JZ, Markel H. Donabedian's lasting framework for health care quality. NEJM. 2016;375(3):205–7.
17. Baldrige Program for Performance Excellence. 2019-2020 Baldrige excellence framework (health care): proven leadership and management practices for high performance. Gaithersburg, MD: U.S. Department of Commerce, National Institute of Standards and Technology; 2019. p. i-58.
18. Lloyd RC. Better quality through better measurement. Orlando, FL: IHI National Forum; 2018.
19. Moen RD, Norman CL. Circling Back: clearing up myths about the Deming cycle and seeing how it keeps evolving. Quality Prog. 2010 (Nov.):22–8. (www.qualityprogress.com).
20. Shewhart WA. Economic control of manufactured product. New York: D. Van Nostrand Company Inc.; 1931.
21. GEP B. Science and statistics. J Am Stat Assoc. 1976;71(356):791–9.
22. Lloyd RC. Navigating in the Turbulent Sea of data: the quality measurement journey. Clin Perinatol. 2010;37(1):101–22.
23. Shewhart WA. Statistical method from the viewpoint of quality control. New York: Dover Publications; 1986.
24. Schultz LE. Profiles in quality: learning from the masters. Quality Resources, a division of The Krause Organization Limited, 1994.
25. Kouzes J, Posner B. The leadership challenge: how to make extraordinary things happen in organizations. San Francisco, CA: Wiley; 2012.
26. Deal TE, Key MK. Corporate Celebration: play, purpose, and profit at work. San Francisco: Berrett-Koehler Publishers, Inc.; 1998.
27. Key MK. The practice of leading. Nashville: M.K. Key; 2013.
28. The W. Edwards Deming Institute. https://blog.deming.org/w-edwards-deming-quotes/large-list-of-quotes-by-w-edwards-deming/. Accessed 15 June 2020. Used with permission from the W. Edwards Deming Institute.

16 Interprofessional Quality Improvement Strategies

Asha S. Payne and Heather Walsh

Introduction

Lauren and Dayna, both physicians, decided to embark on a quality improvement project. They organized meetings, developed a key driver diagram, undertook a thorough analysis of the problem, and decided on the appropriate metrics to measure improvement. After a few months of work, they approached their nursing colleagues, Dory and Chris, to assist with the project. Dory and Chris jumped right in, and the combined team began executing PDSA cycles. Chris helped with collecting data but found it difficult to collect accurate data as she was unfamiliar with the proposed metrics. Though not able to make most of the meetings because she worked the night shift, Dory attended the meetings when she was able. She assisted in executing the PDSA cycles on night shift, but often felt they did not run smoothly as she was not as familiar with the operational aspects of the project. Lauren and Dayna appreciated the help Chris and Dory provided with the project but felt they were not as engaged as they had hoped. In addition, they enjoyed the praise from their senior leadership for creating an interprofessional quality improvement (QI) project. After several months of PDSA cycles, the team achieved improvement in their metrics. Lauren and Dayna eagerly presented the results of the

A. S. Payne (✉) · H. Walsh
Children's National Hospital, Washington, DC, USA
e-tmail: ASpayne@childrensnational.org; HWalsh@childrensnational.org

R. Roberts-Turner, R. K. Shah (eds.), *Pocket Guide to Quality Improvement in Healthcare*,
https://doi.org/10.1007/978-3-030-70780-4_16

work to their senior leadership, eventually publishing a paper to disseminate the findings. What a great example of interprofessional quality improvement! Would Chris and Dory agree? What were the missed opportunities?

Interprofessional Quality Improvement Is More than Working with Another Discipline

In the scenario above, multiple clinical disciplines participated in the QI project, yet they did not have true interprofessional collaboration. Interprofessional collaboration requires sharing, partnership, interdependency, and shared power [1]. In QI, all of the relevant disciplines should actively be involved in each aspect of the project, from assembling the team, determining the scope of the project, conducting PDSA cycles, analyzing the data, and to sharing the results of the work. Lauren and Dayna were the project leaders, and though they eventually partnered with Chris and Dory, there was not true interprofessional collaboration from the beginning. Lauren and Dayna, both physicians, formed the team among themselves; there was no indication of shared power of the project. As such, the above represents a project that Chris and Dory helped with, not a project they owned. Further, there is no indication that Chris' and Dory's perspectives were included in the project, either by updating the key driver diagram or by incorporating additional metrics. Moreover, simply assisting in the execution of the PDSA cycles does not constitute true interprofessional collaboration. There was no interdependency between the physicians and nurses. Lauren and Dayna needed the assistance from Chris and Dory, but there is no indication the converse is true. Finally, there is no indication of shared decision-making or shared power.

Interprofessional Quality Improvement Is More than Doctors and Nurses

Though physicians and nurses are important members of healthcare teams, they are not the only members. Pharmacists, social workers, language interpreters, respiratory therapists, environmental services, information technology, nutrition services, and administrative staff are just a few of the disciplines who may be needed to execute a successful QI project. Each discipline contributes to patient care and the functioning of an organization. In the example above, it is likely that Lauren and Dayna probably could have included at least one other clinical discipline in the work, either pharmacy, social work, or respiratory therapy. The scope of each QI project determines which disciplines should be included, whereas Organizational culture will dictate which clinical disciplines are the easiest to bring together. For some organizations, simply getting two clinical disciplines to meet together is the first step on their interprofessional journey. If that is your organization, start there!

Why Is Interprofessional Collaboration Important for Quality Improvement?

Health care, with all its complexity, is a team sport. Despite this, each clinical discipline learns mostly in silos, with each discipline only perceiving the health-care process from their narrow perspective, without understanding all of the processes impacting patients. Further, understanding complex health-care systems is difficult, and *changing* complex systems is even more so without the input from all disciplines involved. Successful QI work depends on truly understanding all aspects of a health-care system, which cannot happen without all clinical disciplines. As such, limited interprofessional collaboration represents a lost opportunity for understanding health-care complexities and the subsequent improvement that comes from learning these complexities. QI projects are more successful when addressed holistically with the collaboration of interprofessional team members. Look for natural partners: anesthesia and surgery; nurses, physicians, and pharmacists; lactation specialists and nurses. Additional disciplines and service lines can be added as interprofessional collaboration becomes more entrenched in the organization.

Interprofessional Collaboration Is Beneficial to Its Participants

Clinicians, including physicians, nurses, therapists, social workers, and pharmacists, involved in interprofessional quality improvement work cited participating in a highly functioning interprofessional team as the dominant theme for their participation [2]. This indicates that interprofessional collaboration may be a key motivation for many disciplines to engage in QI initiatives. Active interprofessional collaboration in quality improvement projects can streamline processes, improving the delivery of patient care and workflow for staff. Other benefits of interprofessional collaboration include an association with higher teamwork and better inpatient satisfaction scores [3] and better patient outcomes [4]. Additionally, interprofessional collaboration enhances nurse retention through positive practice environments, which include collaborative nurse-physician relationships (e.g., interprofessional involvement in creation of order sets, protocols, interprofessional education activities, and defined roles and responsibilities) [5]. With health care reform, the need for interprofessional teams has never been greater to improve health-care costs, efficiency, and patient outcomes [6].

Every QI Project Does Not Have to Be Interprofessional

Given the complexity of health care, significant or wide-reaching QI projects should be interprofessional collaborations. However, *every* QI project does not have to be interprofessional. Each clinical discipline has skills and perspectives developed within, and improved by, discipline-specific efforts. For example, a QI project aimed at improving the consistency of physician documentation does not require nursing support. Similarly, a QI project to improve nurse retention would not require an interprofessional approach unless poor nurse-physician collaboration was cited as the reason nurses left the organization. If the goal of the QI project is discipline-specific improvement, interprofessional collaboration is perhaps not needed, but if a QI project impacts patients, it likely needs to be interprofessional. Consult with team members to determine the scope of disciplines to be included.

Successful Interprofessional QI Collaboration and Learning

Develop a Culture of Interprofessionalism

Successful interprofessional QI collaboration is driven by an organizational culture that expects and supports interprofessional engagement. In turn, organizational culture is driven by the actions of senior-level and local-level leadership. Consequently, senior-level and local-level leaderships need to authorize, actively support, and engage in, interprofessional collaborations. Individual QI leaders can begin developing a local culture of interprofessionalism by beginning new projects with interprofessional leads. Similarly, existing projects can be reorganized to include interprofessional membership or leadership, as appropriate, being sure to actively incorporate all new participants.

Leadership Support

Local-level leadership for each relevant discipline should be knowledgeable of all interprofessional QI projects. Senior-level support should also be informed, as appropriate. Staff who volunteered (or were appointed) should feel empowered and supported by local leadership to participate in QI activities. Keeping all leaders updated on the progress of initiatives is key. QI project leaders should provide regular updates (presentations, email) to leaders from all the clinical disciplines involved. Getting all leaders together in the same room is preferred, so the QI work can develop and support their interprofessional relationships as well!

Creating Interprofessional QI Teams

Interprofessional QI teams begin with interprofessional leadership. However, interprofessional leadership may not be possible or necessary, depending on the scope of the project. Indeed, the culture of your organization may not be ready for true interprofessional collaboration.

If interprofessional leadership of the team is not possible, then the QI leader should have an eye for creating and fostering an interprofessional team. For example, a QI project to improve antibiotic stewardship may be led by a physician but should be composed of several clinical disciplines. Inviting representatives from other disciplines at the outset of the project is critical. In the scenario at the beginning of the chapter, Laura and Dayna did not involve Chris and Dory until after the project was established. They would have had more engagement and support for the project had they thought to invite them to participate at the outset.

It takes effort to build a high-performing team! Finding engaged staff is the key. Those recruited to join should ideally have experience, or at least a reputation of, working well with others. In addition, appropriate incentives for participating in QI work should be tailored to each clinical discipline. Physicians at academic institutions may be incentivized to participate for either MOC credit, CME credit, or possible publications. Nurses may be encouraged to participate in QI projects if their participation can count towards clinical advancement, promotion, or faculty appointment. Laura and Dayna eventually published the results of the project, but did they include Chris and Dory as authors? Is publication useful for Chris and Dory, or would their careers benefit from another type of reward? Establish the incentive needs of each clinical discipline, including authorship in publications and abstracts, at the beginning of a project or when new members join a preexisting project.

Consider having at least two representatives from each clinical discipline as team members, as this may be necessary to enable regular attendance of each discipline at all team meetings. It is sometimes impossible for a team member to leave clinical care to attend a meeting. Address any possible attendance limitations with each team member at the beginning of their participation.

As mentioned earlier, interprofessional collaborations require sharing, partnership, interdependency, and shared power [1]. Initial team meetings should begin with introductions beyond name and role to begin to build trust and rapport among members. Effective teams identify clear goals, share clarity on roles and responsibilities, communicate openly and honestly, engage all team members, and appreciate diversity within the group. In contrast to multidisciplinary teams where decisions are typically made by one individual, interprofessional teams make decisions jointly [6]. Create equal partnerships among team members through respect and true engagement.

Working in Interprofessional Teams

Coordinating interprofessional QI projects requires careful planning and constant communication. Clinical responsibilities and daily work schedules vary among clinical and nonclinical disciplines. In the scenario at the beginning of the chapter, Chris was not able to attend most of the meetings because of her clinical schedule. Were there any accommodations for her? When planning interprofessional QI meetings, team leaders should consider the schedules of each discipline, scheduling meetings to ensure adequate participation for all members. QI team leaders may need to conduct meetings earlier or later in the traditional workday to account for the demands of shift work. Facilitating coverage for staff members to attend meetings should also be considered. For example, to increase bedside nurse participation in a QI project, consider having an educator or charge nurse cover that nurse's assignment to facilitate meeting attendance. Also, holding shorter, more frequent meetings limits time away from clinical duties. The worst possible times for meetings are between 7 and 8:30 AM and from 3 to 4 PM as this is usually when clinical teams are changing shifts, signing out, or rounding.

Additionally, QI leaders should be aware of the location and accessibility of team meetings. To facilitate attendance from physician and nursing staff on a unit-based project, hold meetings on the unit as opposed to a conference room away from clinical areas. Teleconferencing options should be available for all meetings to encourage staff involvement. To ensure active participation during the meeting, QI team leaders should set an agenda for the meeting. The agenda should be shared in advance. Clear and thorough notes should be taken at each meeting and shared in a timely fashion after the meeting. Of note, email dependence and requirements vary among clinical disciplines. Some staff do not use email as part of their daily work, so email communication may not connect with all team members equally. To account for this, QI leaders or a designee should consider quick, in-person meetings to engage and update those team members as needed.

During meetings, QI leaders should ensure that all professions have the opportunity to share their expertise. If necessary, consider seating arrangements either in an open forum meeting or roundtable. In these meetings, some participant groups may naturally dominate the conversation. An effective QI leader should proactively facilitate sharing from all disciplines. For example, "We haven't heard from the therapists yet. How will this impact you? What has your experience been?"

While the main outcome of the project will be determined by the project charter and leaders, all team members should be involved in the decision-making for additional metrics and the execution of PDSA cycles. When executing PDSA cycles, ensure adequate representation from all disciplines. Also, consider having cross-discipline participation. For example, consider having a pharmacist facilitate the nursing portion of the PDSA cycle. This provides an opportunity for interprofessional learning. During feedback sessions after PDSA cycles, discipline-specific feedback to their peers may yield more useful feedback; however, cross-discipline feedback may elicit more honest responses. Organizational culture and the individual participants will determine which method is best. Experience with QI tools and techniques will also vary among clinical disciplines. Consider incorporating brief educational components to ensure participants have a sufficient understanding of the QI process.

Dissemination of the Work

For public presentations of the work (e.g., abstracts or posters), the presenters should represent as many disciplines as possible. Some disciplines are more comfortable speaking publicly, but all should be provided the opportunity. Senior leadership of all divisions and departments included in the project should be invited to the presentations. For written publications, authorship order should be determined before writing begins. Consider using the acknowledgment section for those who participated in the project but for whom writing credits are not necessary.

If the project is spread to other parts of the organization, make sure each discipline serves as a trainer or resource for the new areas. Any tools created should be shared widely among all the disciplines involved.

Conclusion

In the example presented at the beginning of the chapter, different disciplines were invited to participate in a QI project, but the execution fell short of true interprofessional collaboration. True interprofessional learning and collaboration is more than the participation of different disciplines in a QI project but rather, involves a true partnership through all aspects of a project. The journey to successful interprofessional collaboration begins with leaders and teams understanding where their organizations are on their respective interprofessional journeys. An interprofessional approach to improving complex clinical care systems is difficult, but it creates increased job satisfaction for participants and better experiences for patients. Successful interprofessional collaboration and learning involves following the lead of senior leaders by creating teams with interprofessional leaders and members who truly integrate the strengths of each discipline. QI team leaders need to account for the needs, desires, and limitations of all clinical disciplines. Start with who is willing and available, and expand efforts from there.

References

1. D'Amour D, Ferrada-Videla M, San Martin Rodriguez L, Beaulieu MD. The conceptual basis for interprofessional collaboration: core concepts and theoretical frameworks. J Interprof Care. 2005;19(Suppl 1):116–31.
2. Cumbler EKP, Hagman J. Motivation of participants in an interprofessional quality improvement leadership team. J Interprofessional Educ Pract. 2016;3:5–7.
3. Meterko M, Mohr DC, Young GJ. Teamwork culture and patient satisfaction in hospitals. Med Care. 2004;42(5):492–8.
4. Baggs JG, Schmitt MH, Mushlin AI, et al. Association between nurse-physician collaboration and patient outcomes in three intensive care units. Crit Care Med. 1999;27(9):1991–8.
5. Twigg D, McCullough K. Nurse retention: a review of strategies to create and enhance positive practice environments in clinical settings. Int J Nurs Stud. 2014;51(1):85–92.
6. Eggenberger T, Sherman RO, Keller K. Creating high-performance interprofessional teams. Am Nurse Today. 2014;9(11):12–4.

17 Shared Governance Facilitates Quality Improvement

Gen Guanci

Chapter Content

Data, data everywhere… yet who really owns it? We all know that data is a foundational driver of quality improvement. Leaders are challenged every day to track data specific to their areas. If that data is not meeting organizational expectations, then the leader is charged with improving the data. The leader is now the owner of the data as well as a quality improvement plan yet to be developed.

The leader often spends hours creating a quality improvement plan that she/he is confident will work. The plan is frequently developed with input from other leaders, who may be experiencing the same quality improvement need, are subject matter experts, or will be the individuals educating the staff on the new structures and processes to be followed. The plan gets rolled out to the staff for operationalization, and the data does not improve! As a matter of fact, the staff may not even be operationalizing the plan as they either do not understand the why behind it or do not have the belief the plan will work. Instead of looking at why the plan may not be working or why the staff are resisting, plan owners often

G. Guanci (✉)
Cultures of Excellence, Creative Health Care Management, Bloomington, NM, USA
e-mail: gguanci@chcm.com

R. Roberts-Turner, R. K. Shah (eds.), *Pocket Guide to Quality Improvement in Healthcare*,
https://doi.org/10.1007/978-3-030-70780-4_17

times will revise the plan and include even more details and steps. Thus, the cycle of quality improvement plan failure continues.

A review of the literature for best practices in quality improvement often includes the use of shared governance or shared decision-making as a foundational imperative seen in successful initiatives. Tim Porter-O'Grady, the 1970s pioneer of shared governance, defined it as "a structural model through which nurses can express and manage their practice with a higher level of professional autonomy" [1]. Today, the practice of shared governance or shared decision-making has expanded beyond nursing and is considered an organization-wide leadership model. In their book, *Shared Governance That Works,* authors Guanci and Medeiros share the following definition: "Shared governance is a leadership model in which positional leaders partner with staff in decision-making processes while creating ownership for improvement in practice" [2]. This definition takes shared governance out of the "nursing only" environment and into the inclusive health care environment regardless of what department, area, or specialty leaders and staff work in. In 2016 Porter-O'Grady and colleagues wrote about this evolution into what they termed professional governance [3].

In order to operationalize shared governance, an understanding of the principles and best practices is needed. Shared governance is built on the four (4) principles of partnership, equity, accountability, and ownership [4].

- *Partnership*: Staff members and leaders work together at the unit, department, and organization or system level to improve practice and achieve the best outcomes.
- *Equity*: All contribute within the scope of their roles as part of the team.
- *Accountability*: Staff members and managers share ownership for the outcomes of work; they answer to colleagues, the organization, and the community served.
- *Ownership*: Participants accept that success is linked to how well they do their individual jobs.

In the description of professional governance, Porter-O'Grady and colleagues identify four foundational principles [5]. These principles align and expand on those found in shared governance.

- *Accountability*: This assures that decisions and actions represent the standards of the profession and positively impact the intended client, staff, and organizational outcomes.
- *Professional obligation*: Within the professional role, there are ethical and legal responsibilities that influence practice within the profession, the organization, and the community.
- *Collateral relationships*: This establishes, demonstrates, and expresses equitable interprofessional relationships and interactions.
- *Effective decision-making*: Decisions exercise judgment grounded in the synthesis of evidence-based data to generate alternatives and make informed choices that drive actions and innovation within the profession and the organization.

Whether it be the operationalization of the principles of a shared governance or professional governance model, both supports moving from an "us and them" mindset to a "we" approach to quality improvement.

A belief to address and mitigate is the belief that quality improvement initiatives should be leadership lead. Organizations that have robust shared governance cultures have proven this approach to be incorrect. These organizations see quality improvement initiatives that are adopted quicker and achieve more success in a shorter period of time, and, more importantly, the improvements are sustained over time. Porter-O'Grady states that only 10% of unit- and department-level decisions should be made by the management [5]. To have this occur, a clear understanding of what shared/professional governance is, and what it is not, is needed (Fig. 17.1).

Both the leaders and staff also need to understand and embrace the differences between self-governance, participatory management, and shared governance. As seen in Fig. 17.2, the clear difference is in self-governance, a decision may be made yet never

What Shared Governance Is	What Shared Governance Is Not
Partnership between leaders and staff.	Leader controlling the work
Staff accepting the partnership.	Self-governance
Leaders articulating the expected outcomes	"Us" versus "them" approach
Leaders sharing guardrails for decisions to be made	Leaders abdicating their role
Bi-directional frequent communication between leaders and staff	Not involving leaders in all phases of planning and work
Staff using data to drive their work	Staff only working of "projects" that they choose
Staff accepting the responsibility and accountability for the outcomes of their work	Participatory management
A way to identify future positional leaders	A strategy to support downsizing of leadership
A tenet of professional practice	
A key expression of organizational culture	
A leadership development strategy	

Fig. 17.1 What shared governance is and is not. (Modified from Guanci, G., Medeiros, M., Shared Governance that Works. Used with permission)

operationalized. In participatory management, the staff offer their feedback, yet the leader retains the final decision; in shared governance, the staff make the decision within the guidelines shared by the leader. If a leader is saying "no" when a staff brings a plan to them, then there has clearly been a breakdown and blurring between the models.

The leader's role in a shared governance culture is to be a coach, guide, and developmental facilitator. As a developmental facilitator, the leader uses a longer-term strategy in which the frontline team learns how to facilitate its own processes. The leader helps the team function more effectively on its own – now and in the future – rather than taking charge of the process. Think of it this way: a developmental facilitator helps bring about an outcome by providing indirect or unobtrusive assistance, guidance, or supervision [6].

Parameter	Self-Governance	Participatory Management	Shared Governance
Goals	Staff determine goals without input for leaders	Leaders request input from staff Use of input is optional	Staff are given the responsibility, authority and accountability for decisions
Use of input	Can foster a "they…we"mindset	Leader is not required to use staff input	Leadership and staff activities are interdependent
How decisions are made	All decisions made by work team with no external input or guidance	Final decision lies with leadership, who may accept or reject staff input	Leaders clearly articulate the guidelines for the decision (e.g. we have $10,000 to spend on xx)
Presence of Leader	Absent leader	Hierarchical leader	Servant leader
Where decisions are made	Independent decisions that may never be operationalized	Centralized decision making	Decentralized decision making

Fig. 17.2 Comparison of three styles. (Modified from Guanci, G. Medeiros, M., Shared Governance that Works. Used with permission)

Required Elements to Support Frontline Ownership to Achieve Quality Improvement Outcomes

Up until this point, we have discussed the leader's role in shared governance, but what is the frontline staff's role? How does that role create ownership of data, improvement plans, and the outcomes of those plan?

When we think of who has the most influence on outcomes, it is the person operationalizing or doing the work. It could be the department receptionist greeting the patient that affects whether a patient feels they are being treated with courtesy and respect or not. It is the respiratory therapist that either delivers the breathing treatment on time or not. It is the clinical nurse who either gives the correct medication, at the correct time, to the correct patient or not. The data that leaders review is the autograph of the frontline staff completing the work.

Most frontline staff do not think about data being theirs when, in fact, the drivers of sustained improvement are themselves. If the frontline staff are to own data, they must have a clear understanding of what the data being collected is, what it is telling them, what the desired data target is, and, in some cases, how they compare to other like-type teams. In addition, the frontline staff need to have a clear understanding of responsibility, authority, and accountability (RAA) [7] as it relates to quality improvement ownership.

- *Responsibility*: Clear and specific allocation of duties in order to achieve desired results. It is a two-way street that must be given and accepted, as evidenced by personal ownership and aligned actions.
- *Authority*: This gives the team the right to act and make decisions and is restricted to areas where responsibility is given and accepted. There are four levels of authority (Fig. 17.3) that must be clearly understood, and the specific level of authority must accompany the giving and accepting of the responsibility.
- *Accountability*: The acceptance of the outcomes of the team's work. It is a reflection of the actions, plans, and decision made and is one way to evaluate the effectiveness of these. Figure 17.3 outlines the four levels of authority.

Frontline staff must accept all the three components of the RAA package and not just the responsibility and authority components.

Transparency and sharing of data with frontline staff are the first steps toward ownership. If they do not understand what the

Levels of Authority	
Level 1	Data/Information/Idea Gathering Authority to collect information/data and provide to another who will make the final decision and determine what action will be taken.
Level 2	Data/Information/Idea Gathering + Recommendations Authority to collect information/data, weigh the options and recommend action to be taken to another who will make the final decision.
Level 3	Data/Information/Idea Gathering + Recommendations (Pause to communicate, clarify or negotiate) + Take Action Authority to collect information, apply critical thinking, weigh options, recommend actions, and negotiate the final decision. Includes pausing and collaborating with others before taking action.
Level 4	Act + Inform others after taking action Authority to assess, decide, and act. May follow up and inform another of the actions taken as required by the situation

Fig. 17.3 Four levels of authority. (Used with permission from [8])

data being collected is and what it is telling them, they cannot and will not own it. They will make excuses such as "that's my leader's problem" or "we were having a bad stretch of weather when that happened" or perhaps, in the case of prevalence studies, "that was only 1 day, so not really us."

The way data is presented also has a major impact on understanding. Most staff are not data analysts or experts, so data must be presented in the most basic or simplest form. The manner in which data is shared with frontline staff must be different from the way it is shared with senior leaders. While some may feel this leads to duplication of work, it is well worth the time as it will foster frontline understanding and ownership of data. Visual cues on the desired endpoint, such as an arrow stating "lower is better" or showing the desired direction of the improvement, will go a long way to support frontline staff's understanding.

There is an ancient Chinese proverb that states, "An owner in the business will not fight against it." Shared governance supports this proverb. Using the leadership in shared governance concepts of articulating the expected outcome(s) and the guardrails for plan development, the staff are empowered to craft a plan they are committed to.

Here is an example of how this might look:

- *Problem*: Low "quiet at night" patient satisfaction scores.
- *Expected outcome*: Sustained improvement of associated scores.
- *Quality improvement plan guardrails*: First attempts at problem correction must be in alignment with the organization's policies and procedures and budget neutral.

The frontline team crafts a plan within these articulated guardrails and monitors for improvement, yet only minimal improvement occurs. Upon further discussion with the leadership, additional or new guardrails are established for the team: organization is committing XXX dollars to the purchase of equipment to support the improvement plan, the equipment must come from a vendor within the organization's purchasing/buyer group, and the team is responsible for creating and implementing the education plan associated with the new product.

With these new guardrails, the frontline team can now evaluate equipment options that meet the articulated guardrails. Once they determine what they feel is the best product that meets the articulated guardrails, they share their findings with the leadership. In a shared governance culture, the leadership's response is "thank you, we will order the product while you complete the next phase of crafting the implementation plan." This process fosters commitment to the improvement process as the frontline staff are now the "owner of the business."

What follows are two case studies of how shared governance fostered sustained quality improvement through frontline ownership in the plan.

Interprofessional Case Study

- *Problem and supporting data*: High numbers of reported safety concerns within the hematology/oncology service line. There are 123 reported safety concerns across the hematology-oncology service lines in 1 month, accounting for a rate of 0.115 (safety reports/patient days).
- *Identified etiology*: Lack of structure and processes to facilitate seamless patient care across the inpatient and ambulatory service line areas.
- *Goal*: Reduce the rate of reported safety concerns in all hematology-oncology service line areas.

Performance Improvement Actions

- Interprofessional PI workgroup formed. Disciplines included medicine, frontline staff from nursing, pharmacy, informatics, quality improvement, and operations.
- Assessment of issues through the lens of each discipline completed and analyzed.
- Rapid PDSA cycles to address prioritized issues and ownership for improvement implemented with coaching from quality improvement partners.
- Initial 90-day rapid cycle actions included:
  - Clinic reminder calls to families (operations), nurses assisted with patient placement in the clinic for process flow improvement (nursing), patients with extended infusions were seen by their provider in the infusion center rather than starting in clinic and then going to infusion center

(pharmacy, operations, nursing, and medicine), physician clinic schedule was reviewed and modified to accommodate tumor boards and eliminate patient delays (medicine, informatics, and operations), implemented process of co-signature of chemotherapy orders (informatics, nursing, and pharmacy), and enhanced communication process via daily full-team AM huddles across the service line.

- Second 90-day rapid cycle actions included:
  - Volunteers assigned in clinic for wayfinding and enhancing the patient experience (operations), created visual cues to limit and balance the number of planned procedures and admission across the service line (nursing and operations), implemented enhanced structure chemo delivery to clinic (pharmacy), new process to send chemo orders to pharmacy a day in advance so pharmacy could process medication more timely on day of infusion (nursing and pharmacy), a process developed to ensure that follow-up appointments were made upon hospital discharge (operations), and chart flow remapped in the clinic setting to ensure better patient progression (nursing, operations, and informatics).

- Third 90-day rapid cycle actions included:
  - Follow-up appointment time criteria implemented to improve scheduling and accommodate inpatient admissions versus clinic visit (operations), initiated daily PM huddles across the service line for improved communication and preparation for the next day (medicine, nursing, pharmacy, operations, and informatics), established a direct communication line between the satellite outpatient clinic and main hospital for patients requiring procedures in special procedures unit, (medicine, nursing, operations, and informatics), established a direct communication process for emergency provider coverage in the infusion center (medicine, nursing, and informatics), refined handoff process for patients coming from clinic to special procedures unit including isolation needs and population-specific education to the staff

(nursing), addressed the shift change chemo delivery schedule delay by optimizing communication methods between infusion and hospital pharmacy to decrease shift change chemo delivery delays (operations, pharmacy, nursing, and informatics). Figure 17.4 displays trended outcome data and improvements associated with the interprofessional case study.

Outcome

Nursing Case Study

- *Problem and supporting data*: Increased patient falls on Medical 2 unit. There are 3.55 falls per 1000 patient days.
- *Identified etiology*: Lack of structure and process supporting the proactive addressing of patients at risk for falls.
- *Goal*: Reduce patient falls on Medical 2 unit to below internal target of 1.32 falls per 1000 patient days.

Performance Improvement Actions

- Unit-based shared governance council (UBC) accepted responsibility, authority, and accountability to decrease falls on their unit. UBC members (exclusively frontline nurses) discussed possible evidence-based actions to address issue(s), developed and implemented nurse bedside handoff structure, process, and tool inclusive of introductions of RN to patient, patient safety information, and goals for the shift. All unit staff are educated on the new process and tool by UBC members; continued tracking, trending, and analyzing; and responded to falls data by UBC members. Figure 17.5 displays the trend on the elimination of patient falls as a result of nurse-driven interventions.

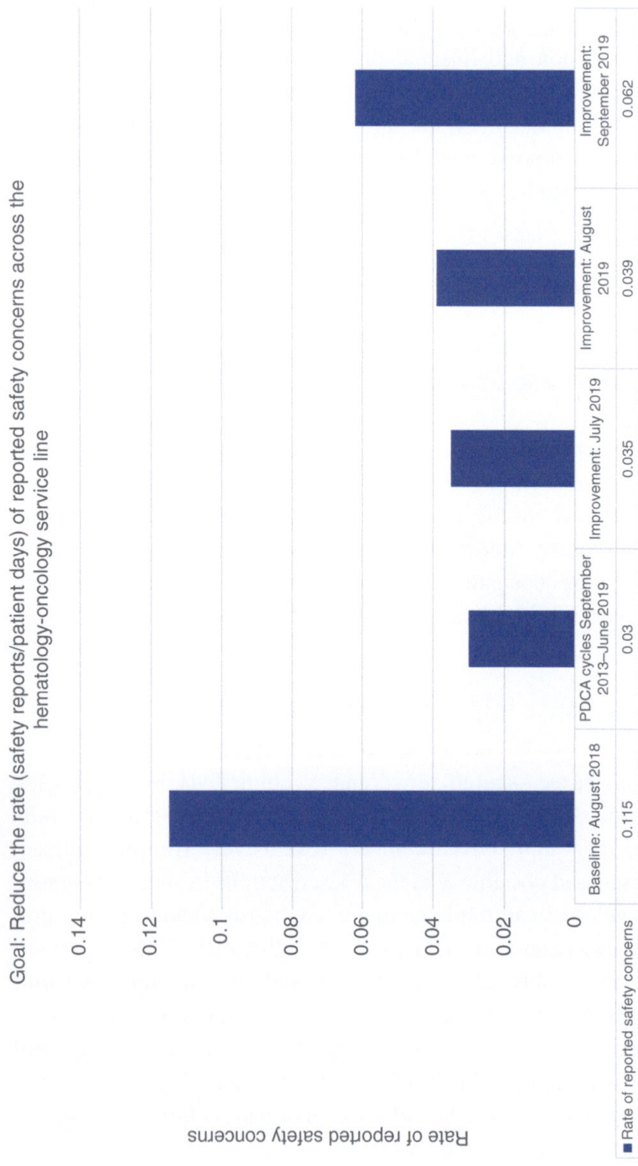

Fig. 17.4 Interprofessional case study outcomes. (Guanci, 2020)

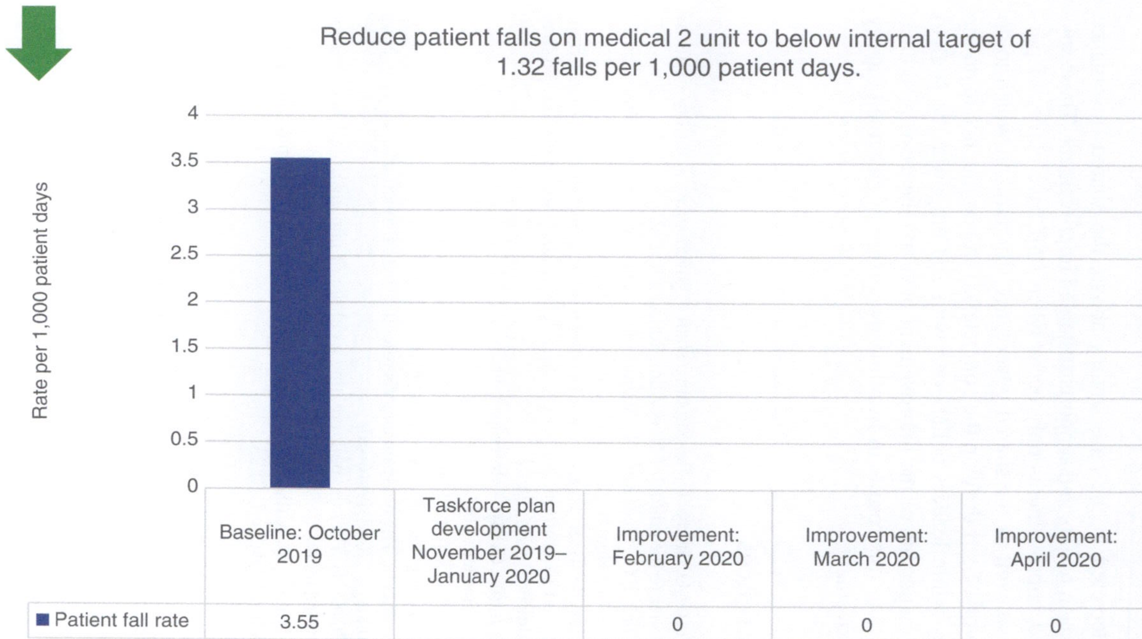

Fig. 17.5 Nursing case study outcomes. (Guanci 2020)

Outcome

As depicted in the case studies above, the shared governance approach fosters and supports sustained improvement. These sustained improvements only occur when staff have clarity of purpose as well as the shared governance structures in which to do the work. Staff develop the competence and confidence to do the work, while leaders collaborate with and empower the staff to take ownership of the improvement plan and the associated data. Together, this results in frontline ownership of sustained quality improvement.

References

1. Porter-O'Grady T. Researching shared governance: a futility of focus [letter to the editor]. J Nurs Adm. 2003;33:251–2.
2. Guanci G, Medeiros M. Shared governance that works. Minneapolis: Creative Health Care Management; 2018. p. 3.
3. Clavelle T, et al. Evolution of structural empowerment: moving from shared to professional governance. JONA. 2016;46(6):308–12. Wolters Kluwer Health, Inc.
4. Porter-O'Grady T. Interdisciplinary shared governance. Sudbury: Jones and Bartlett; 2009.
5. Porter-O'Grady T. Implementing shared governance: creating a professional organization. St. Louis: Mosby; 1992.
6. Guanci G. The nurse manager's role in a shared governance culture. Nurs Manag J. 2018;49:46–50.
7. Guanci G. Feel the pull: creating a culture of nursing excellence. 3rd ed. Minneapolis: Creative Health Care Management; 2016. p. 94–5.
8. Manthey M, Miller D. Empowerment through levels of authority. J Nurs Adm. 1994;24(7–8):23.

18 External Recognition in QI

Jeffrey N. Doucette and Lisbeth D. Fahey

Recognition

Recognition acknowledges achievement of goals, successful outcomes, and quality of care for healthcare organizations. Recognition is awarded at many levels: to the organization, a department, or individuals. External recognition of care and services serves as a public evaluation compared to other similar organizations, which organizations use for self-promotion and marketing. An organization that undergoes a thorough external assessment of structures, processes, and outcomes, through evaluation of best practice implementation, available resources, and results, projects a commitment to quality and improvement. Leaders learn where their organization stands in comparison with others, positive or negative. External survey sponsors recognize excellent performance expressed as rankings or ratings based on these comparative data and information. National surveys repre-

J. N. Doucette (✉)
Thomas Jefferson University Hospitals, Philadelphia, PA, USA
e-mail: jeff.doucette@jefferson.edu

L. D. Fahey
Quality Improvement & Safety, Children's National Hospital,
Washington, DC, USA
e-mail: lfahey@childrensnational.org

R. Roberts-Turner, R. K. Shah (eds.), *Pocket Guide to Quality Improvement in Healthcare*,
https://doi.org/10.1007/978-3-030-70780-4_18

sent a broad spectrum of healthcare organizations. Survey response data serve as a benchmarking tool suitable to foster quality improvement efforts.

Several organizations publish information about healthcare organizations: for-profit companies who use rankings or ratings, such as "honor roll," "best of," or "top" lists, to sell products, publications, and magazines, and some organizations publish data to inform healthcare decision-making. Two organizations that publish rankings and ratings for hospitals are the US News & World Report, a for-profit, and the Leapfrog Group, a nonprofit. These organizations' websites identify their annual rankings/ratings as comprehensive drivers of improvement in safety and quality. According to The Leapfrog Group, their top hospital awards and ratings recognize hospitals with lower error and infection rates and higher quality in measured care areas [1]. The US News & World Report suggests that ranking hospitals and publishing results assist patients in locating the best available care for their condition [2]. Patients and families, applicants for positions, and potential donors consider ratings to determine if the healthcare organization is the right place to receive care, to work, and to provide funding. But hospitals and specialists also use the published information to compare their skills and outcomes with others named in the rankings. Rankings are typically based on quantitative data, such as metrics and outcomes, and on qualitative information, often open-ended questions. These externally reported comparisons drive competition whether intended or not and, like an organizational report card, incentivize improvement and frankly drive improvement and prioritization of resources to improve care delivery.

Federal and state agencies and selected collaboratives publicly report healthcare data that compare generally accepted best practices, processes, and outcomes across hospitals or among clinician groups [3]. These data are generally collected from repositories, such as Medicare. Peer-reviewed articles on the use of survey information and publicly reported data for hospital quality improvement initiatives are available for review. However, the reader cannot conclude that improvement necessarily occurred.

Quality of care initiatives were more likely to show improvement, but it is difficult to determine if improvement in patient safety or patient experience occurred [4].

Surveys

Surveys, in general, are used to collect information and feedback to increase knowledge. Survey design drives the quality of the information received and includes many formats, such as open-ended questions, multiple-choice, multipoint scales or ratings, or ranked preferences. Companies use surveys to learn about consumer preferences, customer satisfaction, or understand employee engagement. Surveys designed to elicit concrete information on the quality or availability of services provided offer a transparent comparison for consumers [5].

External healthcare surveys use a similar approach: collect information on specific aspects of care from organizations or data repositories and report publicly to guide consumer decision-making. Healthcare organizations use survey data to frame and drive improvement initiatives. Survey results provide benchmarking tools for comparing processes and outcomes against those who attain "best of" or "top-ranked" status. Participation in the survey process provides the hospital a self-assessment of internal processes and outcomes and comparison to expected results.

Participation in external surveys varies. The Leapfrog Group Hospital Survey is voluntary, requiring organizations to weigh the benefit and use of information learned from the survey process and results. The US News & World Report "Best Hospitals" adult specialty ranking, published since 1990, includes the American Hospital Association (AHA) member hospitals that fit the survey eligibility requirements. Specialty ranking relies on data available from government and association resources, such as the Centers for Medicare and Medicaid Services patient experience survey (HCAHPS), AHA survey, and specialty group resources. They track patient mortality, volume, staffing ratios, and/or expert physicians' opinions [2]. Their Pediatric Hospital Survey is voluntary, and hospitals must provide a comprehensive survey with general information and extensive data on applicable pediatric specialties to be considered for inclusion.

The US News & World Report Pediatric Hospital Survey and The Leapfrog Hospital Survey rely primarily on self-reported data from submitting organizations. According to the US News & World Reports' online methodology for Best Children's Hospitals, they published the first pediatric rankings based on data in 2007. Since 2008, results have included data on specialty care, with more comprehensive survey data collected annually. Survey questions encompass clinical structures, processes, and outcomes. Data reflect clinical best practices in use, staffing resources, volumes of patients and procedures, and specific clinical outcomes [6]. The Leapfrog Group's website notes that the survey began in 2001 and expanded measures over time [7]. Both survey sponsors retrieve data from external sources when available, such as the Centers for Disease Control External Healthcare Safety Network (NHSN) database and other external data sources with hospitals self-reporting the remainder of information requested. The surveys report that responses are scrutinized using robust processes to ensure valid and reliable data, comparing expected to observed responses and margins for acceptable answers. Survey sponsors request clarification from submitters on any data that are deemed to be out of the expected range for confirmation of responses prior to accepting their survey for publication.

Decisions to participate in voluntary surveys reside at the leadership level as an organizational commitment. Survey completion requires input from numerous content experts in coordination with staff who collects, analyzes, and inputs information into the survey platforms and leaders who validate and verify content prior to submission. To facilitate data collection, robust electronic medical records and information technology platforms are preferred versus manually capturing information from records. Leaders should evaluate the cost of data collection and verification and committed staff time for survey completion in considering participation, determining the return on investment for their organization internally. After survey submission and receipt of published results, leaders determine the best utilization of published results, with information suitable to drive quality improvement initiatives.

Survey Results: Driving Improvement

Once survey results are publicly reported in various formats, organizations have a foundation to improve care using the improvement (QI) process. There are numerous methods to employ in improving quality, such as the Model for Improvement, Lean/Six Sigma, cause analysis, and process mapping. Survey results, as reported, offer basic information and data for organizational response and improvement. The survey sponsors referenced above offer additional opportunities to purchase comparative information: The Leapfrog Group Competitive Benchmarking Reports [8] and US News Hospital Data Insights database [9].

Once the results are available, the QI process begins: review results, compare with benchmarks and your organization's previous results when available, identify improvement opportunities, and prioritize based on importance to patients and the organization. Prioritization should consider the teams who will be charged to make improvements. Microsystems, teams of healthcare members who care for a particular patient population, are an appropriate group to engage in improvement. The US News & World Report Pediatric Hospital Survey results encompass ten specialty groups, and adult hospital surveys rank 16 specialty areas, each inclusive of microsystems. In addition, selected indicators cross specialty groups and encourage the engagement of other professionals in a multidisciplinary improvement approach. Hospital-acquired infections, hand hygiene, and medication processes cross disciplines and microsystems.

Organization support staff, such as patient safety, performance improvement, and patient experience specialists, might round out improvement teams. The organization's expertise to guide and support QI correlates to the capacity and capability to make improvement. Capacity denotes the organization's commitment to educate staff in improvement science to equip them with knowledge and skills to engage in improvement initiatives. Capability refers to building a comprehensive support framework for staff, such as QI and safety department consultants, time to participate in improvement activities, and reinforcement to undertake QI initiatives to improve patient care, safety, or experience.

Well-defined survey data focus the improvement effort, guiding the development of an aim statement that outlines the desired outcome, specific population, and timeline for accomplishment. Microsystem teams identify improvement strategies or key drivers to accomplish the aim: develop processes to improve patient care delivery procedures and outcomes, remove impediments to care access, increase volume, and implement best practices for safe effective care. Measurement is essential to gauge progress with the aim, using benchmarks as comparators.

Achieving improvement within microsystems and across the organization is gratifying for staff, leaders, and the patients who benefit from excellent care, something they expect. Using QI processes as described allows multiple teams to engage in improving care specific to their areas or that will affect care across the continuum. A good starting place is identifying the "low-hanging fruit" or those improvements that are easy to undertake. Hand hygiene is addressed on surveys, with questions about specific compliance measured and processes and practices in place. Once identified as a concern, QI methods might include reviewing and updating policies, evaluating reasons for noncompliance, setting expectations, observing staff compliance, and offering just-in-time education for noncompliance. The outcome is easily measured and compared organization wide. Questions regarding available FTEs may present low-lying solutions if hiring additional resources will improve care and financial resources are available. Reviewing scores for expected numbers of nurses, social workers, or specialty patient/parent educators may justify adding staff. Reviewing current structure and processes may lead to additional specialists, new technologies, or patient support services. Reorganizing structure to allow additional provision of services may be appropriate and improve processes and outcomes. The ability to offer influenza immunizations to specialty clinic patients may be a goal. The structure in place to obtain and store the vaccine needs to be considered with the process of administering the vaccine. Is a licensed staff member available to complete the process? Successful implementation of this QI effort could improve structure, processes, and patient outcomes. Focusing on the process of barcode medication administration scanning compliance engages multidisciplinary teams and potentially reduces medication errors to improve outcomes. The team sets an aim to increase compliance, determines barriers to scanning, develops key drivers to address the barriers, tests potential changes, and measures scanning compliance and medication administration errors to determine outcomes.

Survey questions drive higher-level QI when considering reductions in hospital-acquired conditions, prolonged length of stay, readmissions, or deaths. The QI process and methods remain the same: using data to identify areas for improvement, setting a goal, and implementing the correct actions. The microsystem team likely needs assistance from QI professionals and data analysts. The positive aspect of this type of improvement is that best practices for infection reduction are available for consideration, and small tests of change are easily conducted. Collect and analyze outcome and process data to measure improvement. The QI initiative should be spread and sustained, with the potential to be recognized externally as data are shared.

Other areas for consideration that vary in ease of implementation are specialty accreditation and designation as a Magnet® hospital. Leaders drive decisions to pursue this level of achievement. Rigorous standards must be met, leading to fertile ground for process and outcome QI. Magnet Recognition Program® designation and national organization accreditation favorably impact survey results and are excellent examples of external recognition.

Magnet® Designation

Achieving recognition as a Magnet® designated organization is the highest honor an organized nursing service can achieve. In 1983, the American Academy of Nursing Taskforce on Nursing Practice in Hospitals published their sentinel study, *Magnet Hospitals: Attraction and Retention of Professional Nurses*, which created the evidence base for today's American Nurses Credentialing Center's (ANCC) Magnet Recognition Program [10]. Over the 25-year history of the program, the Commission on Magnet Recognition (COM), the governing body of the Magnet program, has increasingly raised the bar for the performance of Magnet-designated organizations. Initially focused on the 14 forces of magnetism, factors found to influence recruitment and retention, the Magnet standards have evolved an outcomes-based model that are essential to a culture of excellence and innovation in nursing practice [10]. The Magnet standards are rooted in a strong, independent scientific base that spans 20 years of research and development.

The Magnet model consists of five components: structural empowerment; exemplary professional practice; new knowledge, innovation, and improvements; and transformational leadership all of which underpin the final component, empirical outcomes. The model acknowledges that global issues in nursing and healthcare impact the five Magnet domains (Fig. 18.1). Each of the five

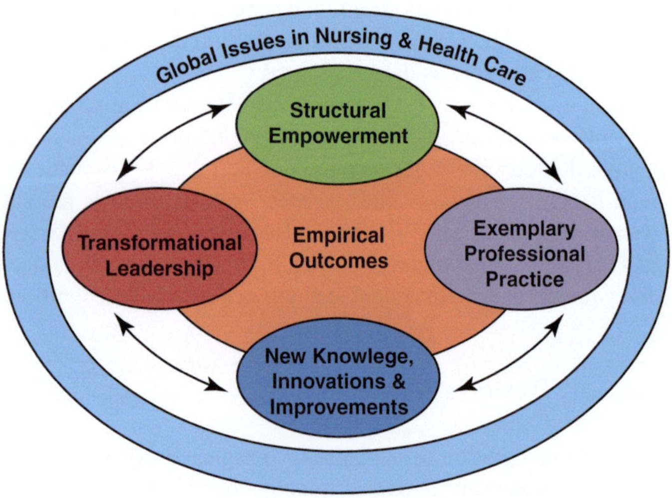

Fig. 18.1 ANCC Magnet® model. The Magnet model consists of five components: structural empowerment; exemplary professional practice; new knowledge, innovation, and improvements; and transformational leadership all of which underpin the final component, empirical outcomes

components has a series of sources of evidence (SOE) that must be met by the applicant organization to achieve Magnet designation. Once achieved, the designation period is 4 years, during which time designated organizations will participate in an interim monitoring report and begin the redesignation process.

Before applying for Magnet designation, organizations should complete a gap analysis based on the current Magnet application manual standards. Tools and resources for organizations considering Magnet designation are available from the ANCC Magnet Recognition Program website. It is imperative that organizations understand the eligibility requirements, the Magnet model, and the required sources of evidence before beginning the application process.

The process to achieve Magnet designation consists of four major elements: application, submission of documents, a site visit, and Commission on Magnet decision. The application is the first step and declares the organization's intent to submit written documents. During this phase, organizations will submit documentation regarding the organizational structure, qualifications of the chief nursing officer (CNO), and other nurse leaders, as well as other documents establishing the eligibility of the organization. Following the application, organizations will prepare and submit documents, the second phase of the designation process. This stage of the process can take from several months up to a year or more depending on the readiness of the organization at the time of application. The documents contain examples of how the organization meets the SOE under each of the components of the Magnet model and tells the story of the contributions of nurses to the empirical outcomes achieved by the applicant. The requirements for the documents are very specific and must be followed clearly and precisely to be appropriately evaluated and scored by the appraisal team. Once the documents are submitted, they are reviewed and scored by an independent appraisal team. The results of the document submission phase could be one of the three following scenarios: the document does not meet the standards, and the application process ends; the document meets the minimum thresholds, but additional documentation is required; or the document meets the standards, and the organization advances to the next phase of the appraisal process, the site visit. Organizations that required additional documentation are given a one-time opportunity to provide additional examples and data in order to move to the site visit phase. The site visit is the highlight of the journey for many organizations on the Magnet journey. The visit is conducted by the same team of appraisers who reviews and scores the document. The purpose of the site visit is to clarify, amplify, and verify the contents of the written document. Once the site visit concludes, the appraiser team submits a written report to the COM, who makes the final determination of designation status.

Since the inception of the Magnet program, numerous studies have examined the impact of implementing the various elements of the Magnet model on the organization. Work culture, retention, nurse-sensitive outcomes, and patient satisfaction are a few of the areas which have been widely examined in the literature. The strong scientific basis of the Magnet Recognition Program continues to evolve as the program itself continues to grow. Once a modest program centered on hospitals in the United States, the Magnet Recognition Program has grown to over 500 designated hospitals worldwide.

Recognition, such as a Magnet Recognition Program®-designated organization, Leapfrog Top Hospital, or US News Best Hospital, represents a beginning, not an end, to improving quality. As you dive into survey data to determine what and how to improve, many opportunities may emerge. Over time, QI efforts mature and result in overall performance improvement, followed by recognition at many levels: internal and external. But also consider that other organizations are attempting to improve quality with the same consequences of better outcomes and improved ratings and rankings, pushing the bar for the quality of care and external recognition higher. The cycle continues. Quality improvement in clinical outcomes, processes, and structures readies the organization for the next survey submission. Quality improvement involves everyone working together to attain excellent results and positive outcomes. A top survey ranking or rating externally recognizes that an organization values and provides the best quality patient care. In the end, the winners are the patients receiving top-notch care and the staff choosing to work in externally recognized healthcare organizations.

References

1. Top Hospitals [Internet]. The Leapfrog Group. 2020 [cited 15 May 2020]. Available from: https://www.leapfroggroup.org/ratings-reports/top-hospitals
2. FAQ: How and Why We Rank and Rate Hospitals [Internet]. US News & World Report. 2020 [cited 3 June 2020]. Available from: https://health.usnews.com/health-care/best-hospitals/articles/faq-how-and-why-we-rank-and-rate-hospitals
3. Public Reporting as a Quality Improvement Strategy: A Systematic Review of the Multiple Pathways Public Reporting May Influence Quality of Health Care | Effective Health Care Program [Internet]. Effectivehealthcare.ahrq.gov. 2020 [cited 28 May 2020]. Available from: https://effectivehealthcare.ahrq.gov/products/public-reporting-quality-improvement/research-protocol
4. Fung C, Lim Y, Mattke S, Damberg C, Shekelle P. Systematic review: the evidence that publishing patient care performance data improves quality of care. Ann Int Med [Internet]. 2008 [cited 20 May 2020];148(2):111. Available from: https://doi.org/10.7326/0003-4819-148-2-200801150-00006
5. Brogan N. Industry Voices—6 types of healthcare surveys that can improve patient experiences [Internet]. FierceHealthcare. 2020 [cited 15 May 2020]. Available from: https://www.fiercehealthcare.com/practices/industry-voices-6-types-healthcare-surveys-can-improve-patient-experiences
6. Methodology: U.S. News & World Report Best Children's Hospitals 2020–21 [Internet]. Copyright © 2020 U.S. News & World Report, L.P. Data reprinted with permission from U.S. News. 2020 [cited 20 May 2020]. Available from: https://health.usnews.com/media/best-hospitals/BCH_methodology_2020-21.pdf
7. History [Internet]. Leapfrog. 2020 [cited 15 May 2020]. Available from: https://www.leapfroggroup.org/about/history
8. Competitive Benchmarking [Internet]. Leapfrog. 2020 [cited 15 May 2020]. Available from: https://www.leapfroggroup.org/ratings-reports/competitive-benchmarking
9. Hospital Data Insights [Internet]. Hdi.usnews.com. 2020 [cited 19 June 2020]. Available from: https://hdi.usnews.com
10. American Nurses Credentialing Center. 2019 Magnet® Application Manual. ISBN-13: 978-0615844251.

Abbreviations and Definitions

Abbreviations

ACA	Apparent cause analysis
AHRQ	Agency for Healthcare Research and Quality
ANA	American Nurses Association
ANCC	American Nurses Credentialing Center
API	Associates in Process Improvement
ARCC	Ask, request, concern, chain of command
ASHP	American Society of Health-System Pharmacists
BPEP	Baldrige Performance Excellence Program
C. diff	*Clostridioides difficile*
CAUTI	Catheter-associated urinary tract infections
C-Chart	Count chart
CDC	Centers for Disease Control and Prevention
CIN	Clinically integrated network
CL	Center line on a control chart
CLABSI	Central line-associated bloodstream infection
CME	Continuing medical education
CMS	Centers for Medicare & Medicaid Services
COM	Commission on Magnet
CQI	Continuous quality improvement
CVC	Central venous catheter
DART	Days away, restricted, or transferred
DMAIC	Define, measure, analyze, improve, control

R. Roberts-Turner, R. K. Shah (eds.), *Pocket Guide to Quality Improvement in Healthcare*,
https://doi.org/10.1007/978-3-030-70780-4

EHR	Electronic health record
ESS	Employee staff safety
FMEA	Failure modes and effects analysis
HAC	Hospital-acquired condition
HAI	Hospital-acquired infection
HCAHPS	Hospital consumer assessment of healthcare providers and systems
HRO	High reliability organization
HSOPS	Hospital survey on patient safety culture
IHI	Institute for Healthcare Improvement
IOM	Institute of Medicine
IR	Incident report; also known as safety event report
IT	Information technology
LCL	Lower control limit
LOR	Levels of reliability
MAR	Medical administration record
MB-CLABSI	Mucosal-barrier central line-associated bloodstream infection
MFI	Model for improvement
MOC	Maintenance of certification
MUE	Medication-use evaluation
NAHQ	National Association for Healthcare Quality
NCC MERP	National Coordinating Council for Medication Error Reporting and Prevention
NDNQI	National Database Nursing Quality Indicators
NPSF	National Patient Safety Foundation
P-Chart	Proportion chart
PDSA	Plan-do-study-act
PHI	Preventable harm index
PI	Performance improvement
PI	Pressure injury
PPE	Personal protective equipment
PU	Pressure ulcer
QBS	Quality as a business strategy
QI	Quality improvement
RAA	Responsibility, authority, and accountability
RCA	Root cause analysis

RPN	Risk priority number
S-Chart	Standard deviation chart
SCS	Safety culture survey
SER	Safety event report
SMART	Specific, measurable, achievable, realistic, and timely
SOE	Sources of evidence
SOI	Science of improvement
SOPK	System of profound knowledge
SPC	Statistical process control
SPS	Solutions for patient safety
STAR	Stop, think, act, review
TAT	Turnaround time
TCR	Therapeutic class review
TRIR/TRCR	Total recordable incident rate or total case incident rate
UBC	Unit-Based Shared Governance Council
UCL	Upper control limit
UE	Unplanned extubation
UPC	Unit Practice Council
X-bar-S Chart	Average and standard deviation chart

Definitions

Accident	An unplanned, unexpected event, usually with an adverse consequence
Adverse event	Injury caused by medical care
Benchmarking	Setting goals and developing comparisons based on what has been achieved by others
Blood and body fluid exposures	When a patient's blood or body fluids come into contact with a healthcare provider's skin or mucous membranes such as the eyes, nose, or mouth
Closed loop communication	A communication technique that ensures a message sent by the "sender" was received, interpreted, and understood by the receiver
Corrective action	An action the manager(s) or organization intends to implement to reduce or prevent future repeat events

Electronic health record (EHR)	Computerized system to document, store, and display patient health data and medical records. Used in healthcare settings by clinical and administrative staff to manage healthcare for individual patients and across populations
Error	An unintended act that produces an undesirable result or significant potential for an undesirable result
Extent of condition	The likelihood that given a certain set of conditions that resulted or potentially resulted in harm
Fall	A sudden, unintentional descent that results in the individual coming to rest on the floor, on or against some other surface, on another person, or on an object
Four levels of authority	The level at which a group has the authority to make a decision
Hazards	Events, actions, or things that can cause harm
Health information technology (IT)	Refers broadly to electronic health records and related applications and devices used in the delivery of healthcare services
Hospital-acquired condition	A condition that occurs during hospitalization (or medical care)
Hospital-acquired infection	An infection occurring during hospitalization (or medical care)
Incidence	A measurement used to track the rate that a condition occurs during a specified period of time within a population
Incidents	Occurrences or events that have or could lead to undesirable results
Incident report/ occurrence report	Form (usually electronic) used to communicate the occurrence of a clinical safety event (which may be a near miss, know complication, precursor event, or serious safety event) to internal stakeholders. The occurrence information is used to promote appropriate event response and to promote patient safety and quality improvement going forward
Known complication	An adverse outcome supported in the literature as a potential risk related to a procedure, treatment, or test that is not present before the patient care encounter and occurs as a result of patient care

Lateral integration	The process of issue identification, resolution, and spread across the organizational continuum to ensure that lessons learned and corrective actions are shared with those other areas to prevent repeat events
Near miss safety event	A deviation from accepted practice standards that does not reach the patient. The error is caught by detection or inadvertently
Overexertion injuries	Caused by directing excessive physical effort at an object (lifting, pulling, carrying, throwing), repetitive motion (typing, using tools or instruments), and free bodily motion (bending, crawling, twisting, kneeling)
Principles of shared governance	Partnership, equity, accountability, and ownership
Precursor safety event	A deviation from accepted practice standards that reaches the patient. The error results in minimal to non-detectable harm
Preventable Harm Index	A tool used to track and trend harm and errors
Prevalence	An epidemiological measure of how often a condition occurs within a population. It measures how much of the population is affected by a particular condition at a particular point in time
Quality improvement plan guardrails	Limits or criteria that must be met when creating a quality improvement plan
Risk	The possibility of loss or injury
Safe lifting	Proper use of lifting techniques and safe patient handling equipment to decrease injuries
Serious safety event	A deviation from accepted practice standards that reaches the patient. The error results in moderate to severe harm or death
Shared governance	A leadership model in which positional leaders partner with staff in decision-making processes while creating ownership for improvement in practice
Sharps and needlestick injuries	Injuries to the skin that are caused by sharp instruments and hollow-bore needles (lancet, scalpels, glass, hypodermic needles, butterfly needles, suture needles, syringe needles, IV catheter stylets) that accidentally penetrate the skin in a healthcare setting

Slip	A loss of friction between an individual's footwear and the floor
Solutions for patient safety	The leading pediatric improvement collaborative
Trip	A physical obstacle like a loose tile, objects in a walk path, cracked sidewalk, or floor surface that prevents an individual from completing a step
Workplace violence	Any physical assault, verbal abuse, or threatening disruptive behavior in the workplace can occur anywhere, but certain industries such as healthcare are prone to increase physical and verbal violence from patients, visitors, and employees

Index

R. Roberts-Turner, R. K. Shah (eds.), *Pocket Guide to Quality Improvement in Healthcare*,
https://doi.org/10.1007/978-3-030-70780-4

MIX
Papier aus verantwortungsvollen Quellen
Paper from responsible sources
FSC® C105338

If you have any concerns about our products,
you can contact us on
ProductSafety@springernature.com

In case Publisher is established outside the EU,
the EU authorized representative is:
Springer Nature Customer Service Center GmbH
Europaplatz 3, 69115 Heidelberg, Germany

Printed by Libri Plureos GmbH
in Hamburg, Germany